To: Doris

# Sister Feelgood

" WE HOPE THIS
LITTLE BOOK CAN
ADD A BOUNCE
To YOUR STEP
ALL YEAR ~~LONG~~ "

Fr: WENDY
&
BARON

CHRISTMAS
2000 -

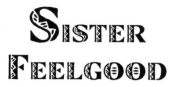

# Sister Feelgood

A Year of Health and
Fitness for Our Bodies
and Our Souls

Donna Marie Williams

Three Rivers Press
New York

To *mi familia*

Published by Three Rivers Press, a division of Crown Publishers, Inc., 201 East 50th Street, New York, New York 10022. Member of the Crown Publishing Group.

Random House, Inc. New York, Toronto, London, Sydney, Auckland
http://www.randomhouse.com/

THREE RIVERS PRESS and colophon are trademarks of Crown Publishers, Inc.

Printed in the United States of America

Design by Mercedes Everett

Library of Congress Cataloging-in-Publication Data is available upon request.

ISBN 0-517-88488-7

10 9 8 7 6 5 4

# ACKNOWLEDGMENTS

This book might never have been written had it not been for the support and love of friends and family. First and foremost, thank you, George and Hyacinth Williams, for being the greatest parents on the planet (maybe in the universe).

Laura and Janice Williams, my blood sisters and best friends, listened to me rant and rave about diet industry conspiracies, big hips, and the Black men–Black women thing. Bertha Baskin and Sheila Jones, co-workers and sisterfriends par excellence, taught me the value of having high expectations. Not only did I apply their lessons to the writing of this book, the concept has changed my entire life.

I am especially grateful to the two highly competent, strong, progressive Black women who made *Sister Feelgood* possible—Denise Stinson, my literary agent, and Carol Taylor, my editor. When the sisterhood gets together on a project, watch out.

And finally, Michael and Ayanna, my wonderful, smart, energetic children, were truly good during the writing of this book. They gave me the space I needed, and I will be forever grateful. They're the reasons why I try so hard.

**M**y good body used to be fat when I was a girl—or so I thought. I now long for that brick house of a body. I was stacked and didn't know it. All I knew was that my round, developing, African-woman body was getting a lot of male attention, and, being painfully shy, I didn't know how to handle it. Nor did I know how to deal with the fact that I just didn't have a ballerina body. I had danced since nine years old, and as I grew older, I began to look voluptuous in my leotards rather than artistically lean and bony. My legs and breasts were simply too big. The message I received was that my round hips and tiny waist were for a man's hands, not Carnegie Hall. I was fifteen years old when I was told at an audition that the only way I could be a dancer was to lose weight. Well, I had tried that before, and had fainted a couple of times from the attempt.

I wish I had known back then that my body was beautiful. To tell the truth, I wish I had that body right now, because today, my good body really is fat. Not fat, really. Kind of pillowlike—soft, cushy. My real body is about 70 pounds lighter than what registers on the scale. Beneath this extra flesh, I can feel its swells and curves. This extra flesh is a nuisance. It weighs heavy on my soul.

I wish I had known back then that my body was beautiful, but the challenge is to know it now. I know I'm not alone. Even though we Black women have different body stories to tell, most of us share a nagging dislike for the way our bodies have responded to PMS, babies, menopause, illness, stress, grief, and time. We also share a guilt because we know deep down that we've allowed the flab to happen.

I wrote this book as a selfish act of love, although I didn't know I loved myself when I began writing. I've wanted to lead a healthy lifestyle for a long time now, but I couldn't find a book, tape, or class that realistically and honestly addressed my needs as a Black woman and a single mother. The problem, I've come to realize, is that health is not an integral part of our culture. Health-conscious vegetarians and exercisers, for example, are viewed with suspicion by our people. They are called "health nuts" or "white acting."

Look at our communities. There are many more liquor stores in our neighborhoods than health food stores. And who among us hasn't gone to the white people's neighborhood at least once to buy fresh meats and produce at reasonable prices? Religion has become so divisive among our people that many of us *will not* learn from the healthy eating practices of "radical cults," such as the Seventh-Day Adventists, Muslims, and Hebrew Israelites. Our barbecues, house parties, and family reunions are about alcohol, cigarettes, fattening foods, and unprotected sex.

The purpose of *Sister Feelgood* is to awaken a sick and sleeping giant. Over the course of the next 365 days, you'll read about some of the ways we Black women lead the nation in sickness, depression, and death—but please do not use this information to maintain a victim status. That would be a blaspheming of the book's purpose. Black folks can no longer luxuriate in ignorance and denial. The sins of the mothers and fathers are being visited upon our children. Our children are eating greasy potato chips for breakfast and McDonald's for lunch and dinner. We cannot allow this to continue.

So, out of necessity, this book takes the approach that health must be an individual and a communal endeavor. It is our responsibility as Black women—the primary nurturers, teachers, cooks, and caregivers of the community—to educate ourselves about healthy living.

Commit the next 365 days of your life to creating a healthy lifestyle. Immerse yourself in health. Work with this book. Let me give you my testimony. I won't lie to you and say that I've lost 100 pounds and have 80 percent lean muscle mass (although I'm working on it). I can say that for the first time in my thirty-six years, I actually love myself just as I am—flab, sag, and all. I have learned to make health a priority and put weight loss into perspective. I have meaningful work. I have good friends and a great family. My life is so full, it overflows at times. Amazingly, the weight is slowly beginning to come off, after all these years.

I've tried to lose weight many times over the past couple of decades. I now realize I was putting the cart before the horse. The most important lesson I've learned is that once you get your soul healed, the body healing will certainly follow. That's what *Sister Feelgood* is all about. I'm a witness.

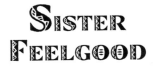

# SISTER
# FEELGOOD

# DAY 1

*"I feel good!"*

Sisters, let's dedicate this next year to feeling good. No more moaning and groaning and crying and whining about fat and aches and pains. It's time to take action. Our success in creating a healthy, fit lifestyle absolutely depends on a powerful belief in our ability to manifest. Don't let past failures undermine your belief in your own power. Some of us have been playing at the diet game for so long that it's easy to remember the failures while forgetting the *sheer tenacity* it has taken to keep on trying. Think about all the roadblocks you've experienced over the years: illness, pregnancy, stress on the job, stress in relationships, grief, the fact that you're a woman and your body has been designed to retain fat. Hey, how about plain and simple hunger? That you have not succeeded says nothing about your worth as a human being—*the fact that you keep trying does.* The ability to lose weight is within you, so you must never lose the faith. If "faith is the substance of things hoped for, the evidence of things not seen," then you are already slim, fit, and healthy. Keep the faith!

*Doubts have no place in my thinking and feeling. I believe in my power to manifest a healthy, fit body!*

# DAY 2

*"Girl, I'm going on a diet this year. No, for real."*

Do we really want to go through *that* exercise in futility: the New Year's Resolution List? And which resolution tops everyone's list? Weight loss. Let's consider a new approach. Throw the list in the garbage. Now, instead of resolving to do something tomorrow, use the day to feel and visualize the changes you want to make in your body and your life *today*. Close your eyes and feel the pounds melt off your body. See the new you in your mind's eye. Imagine yourself in new, outrageous clothes. See your hair styled in a different way. Now go to your kitchen and throw out one food item that's no good for you, just one. Go outside and walk briskly around the block. The point of all this is to make the beginning of the new year a time for action. Don't waste the day on writing the same tired list you wrote last year. Instead, start the year off on a good foot. You'll set a powerful, positive tone for the next 363 days.

*I commit myself to action today!*

# DAY 3

*Diet strategies that make you go HUH?*

Strategy #1: Grazing. Right, like a cow. This diet strategy replaces our three squares a day with five, even six, *small* snacklike meals throughout the day. The idea is that constant eating will keep your metabolism up and appetite down. Strategy #2: Eat a ton, weigh less. This diet strategy relies on low-fat, high-energy, carbohydrate-rich foods like pasta, vegetables, and fruit for its success. Strategy #3: Programmed eating. Overeaters Anonymous, Weight Watchers, and Jenny Craig advocate three strict calorie-controlled meals and two snacks a day. Behavior modification is stressed. Strategy #4: The Honorable Elijah Muhammad prescribed one vegetarian meal a day, with periods of ritual fasting. Clearly, there is no shortage of plans. The question is, which one is best for you? The secret to success is balance, consistency, and an understanding of yourself—your style of eating, your biorhythms, your moods.

*I will choose the eating program
that's right and healthy for me.
Better yet, I will create my own
program.*

# DAY 4

*The lonely woman has a hungry heart.*

When Black women get together to talk, the conversation inevitably jerks toward men. We may have unique stories to tell about our fathers, brothers, husbands, sons, and lovers but we sing the same sad songs. Why won't they talk to us? Why do they leave? Why are they so strange? We commiserate on the phone, or worse, we eat boxes of doughnuts, bags of potato chips, and gallons of ice cream. What's a lonely woman to do? Well, begin by not looking at your sister friendships as poor seconds to your relationships with men. They each have their place, and as we know, if a relationship with a man falls apart, it's the sisterfriend who listens and consoles us. Second, start moving. Exercise is a great antidote to depression, releasing all those feelgood endorphins in the brain. Most important, if you've done all you can do and your relationship still does not make you happy, maybe it's time to move on.

*I will eat to satisfy hunger, not to push down emotions.*

# DAY 5

*I love my neck.*

How do I love my neck? Let me count the ways. I love
my neck because it holds up my head. I love my neck
because I can wrap designer silk scarves and hang beautiful necklaces from it. I love my neck because it contains everything I need for swallowing good, healthy
food. It may be a little thicker than it used to be, but it
works just as well as it ever did. Because our necks are
so close to our brains, stressful thinking makes it hurt
at times. Well, maybe. Truth is, we neglect our necks,
take them for granted. Today we're going to love our
necks for bearing the pressure of holding up our heads
so well. First, take out your prettiest neck accessory and
wear it today. Second, sit up straight and tall, and carry
yourself regally, like the African queen you are. Third,
if the back of the neck hurts from stress, roll it, tilt it,
stretch it, knead it. Roll it around and around. Tilt it
from side to side. Now, doesn't that feel better?

*I will bless my neck throughout the
day for doing such fabulous work.*

# DAY 6

*Will builder: Boycott food for a day.*

Every once in a while, it's a good idea to go totally without food. No, you won't die. Fasting on water or pure fruit and vegetable juices will clean you out and strengthen your will, not to mention your body. Fasting will also give your digestive system some peace. Fasting can be a very intimidating experience, but it needn't be. Anticipating some of the initial discomforts should help calm your fears. For example, don't be surprised when, on the first day, you experience headaches, nausea, or other physical discomforts. This is your body cleansing itself of toxins. Drinking prune juice a day or two prior to fasting may help. The psychological discomforts, on the other hand, may be a bit more disconcerting. Part of the pleasure of eating is in the chewing. But the mind's ability to adapt to even this, the absence of food, is remarkable—and a blessing.

*A little sacrifice is good for building my will. I will try fasting today, from dawn till dusk or for just one meal, whatever I can manage.*

# DAY 7

*"I'm fat." "My breasts sag." "My thighs look like cottage cheese." "I look like I'm pregnant." "Is that my butt?"*

Making peace with our bodies in this Age of Barbie is an uphill battle for those of us who do not fit the mold. The Black woman's struggle is particularly keen, given the ample ways our bodies refuse to conform to the standard. The prelude to inner peace is the calling of a truce to the war raging within our souls. Cease firing criticisms at your body today. Stop it right now. Your body is precious, has carried you through thick and thin. Make peace with your body. Lavish praise on your body. Look in the mirror and tell your naked body that it's a beautiful body. Sink deeply into a tub of bubbles. Get a massage. Your toes deserve a pedicure. Learn to love your body. Exercise it. Pamper it. As you give your body much a deserved rest, it will reward you with health, strength, and vitality.

*Today I will chill and make peace*
*with my body.*
*It's a good beginning.*

# DAY 8

*It is written that Black folks don't plan beyond next week, much less twenty years down the road.*

One of the weaknesses we Black people must collectively correct is our failure to make and follow through on our goals. We are a jazzy people, a go-with-the-flow type folk, which is fine, but unless you've got a plan, you're going to flow right on out to nowhere. The process of defining and writing down your goals is a tool of empowerment. To strengthen our communities we must create short- and long-term goals. To restore our bodies, we must have a short-term goal that defines our desire to reach our destination of health and fitness and a long-term goal that defines a maintenance plan. Write down your body goals and tape them everywhere so you won't forget—on your bedpost, on your refrigerator, on your mirrors. Tomorrow we'll discuss how to manifest those goals.

*I have a vision! I know*
*where I want to go.*
*I will document my goals.*

# DAY 9

*Plan to work, and work to plan.*

Goals are great for defining the vision of where you want to go in life, but *how* you will get there is critical to making your goals a reality. Goals are nothing without a plan of action to move you from point A to point B. Determine first where you are—your health status (now would be a good time for a checkup), your weight, and your fitness level (can you walk briskly without passing out?). Look at the areas that need strengthening and determine how to proceed. If you can't walk and talk at the same time, it's time to start exercising. Short of breath all the time, but you're still smoking? You know what to do—quit! Much too heavy, and you know it? Do your research. Look into the many food programs (diet is now a bad word) and determine which one would be best for you.

*I will create my health and fitness
action plan today!*

# DAY 10

*The devil made me do it.*
—GERALDINE (A.K.A. FLIP WILSON)

When we first started hearing about the widespread occurrence of heart disease in America, we were told that we had to reduce the risk factors in our immediate environment that were causing the disease. Risk factors, like the devil, make us do bad when we want to do good. They also increase the possibility of harm. Our communities abound with risk factors: alcohol and tobacco billboards, pollution, landfills, and fast-food joints. Our refrigerators are full of junk food, alcohol, and lard. Our homes encourage sedentary living, with a TV in every room. On the whole, we have not yet internalized the behaviors and beliefs that would protect us from obesity, sickness, and disease. Granted, your environment can never be completely risk-free, but you can begin to eliminate those things (and people) that sabotage your efforts to become healthy and free.

Nothing *is going to
sabotage my eating and exercise
program today.*

# DAY 11

*"Girl, it's a rough world out there. I got to protect myself."*

Wouldn't it be great if we lived in a world without temptation? No lasagne commercials, no skinny models to piss us off, no uncooperative mates and friends—just peace and love. Oh well. Truth is, temptations specifically designed to throw us off our program are lurking behind every corner, candy wrapper, and women's magazine cover. But we can fight. We must take responsibility for meeting our goals. That means building support mechanisms into our life. Look for a support group, a new job if need be, new friends. Get the kids to buy in to what you're doing for yourself. Tell them what you need them to do and say. Don't have junk food lying around the house. Try keeping fresh fruit around instead. For all the factors that you can control, take charge. And for all those that you can't, go with the flow.

*I am going to protect myself from anything that would undermine my progress today.*

# DAY 12

*What is a carbohydrate?*

There are two types of carbohydrates—simple sugars and complex starches—and they are everywhere: in some dairy products, legumes, nuts, seeds, beverages, vegetables, grain products, fruits, and cereals. Our bodies need carbohydrates for fuel. The digestive system breaks down the carbohydrates in food into glucose, which is then distributed to the muscles for energy. Carbohydrate-rich foods are diet staples because they are abundant and cheap (compared to meat, poultry, and fish). We use them to stretch our meals and, best of all, they make us feel full. *Caution:* Following the trip to the muscles, the glucose then parks in the liver and fat cells. Mainstream women's magazines talk a lot about eating pasta, beans, and baked potatoes, and it's OK for you to take their advice if you're exercising regularly and if you do not have a sensitivity to carbohydrates. Otherwise, you're going to have a lot of big, energized fat cells on your thighs!

*Like my mama used to say,*
*moderation in all things is the key*
*to health and happiness.*

# DAY 13

*The road to health is paved with knowledge.*

If you're really serious about improving the overall health of your body, you've got to do your homework. This is a critical step that should not be given a pass. Our people are perishing for a lack of knowledge; Black people lead the races in this country in disease and death rates. And for what? If information is power, and if information is plentiful, then we have no excuse. Go into any library, book or grocery store and take your pick. There are tons of information on nutrition, exercise, and health. Check out the new health-oriented cooking shows on TV. Talk to people who have made great strides in their own programs. Once armed with knowledge, begin to apply what you know. A great mind once said, "Faith without works is dead." No truer words have been spoken. Let's get busy.

*I'm going to do my homework
today. I'm going to
study ways to improve my body.
Then I'll apply it.*

# DAY 14

*"Girl, them pounds ain't nothing but stress weight."*

The word *stress* has become our favorite catchall word for whatever ails us. Got an ache? It's from stress. Gained (or lost) some weight? It's from stress. Our understanding of stress as underlying most of our body's predicaments is right in line with emerging research theory. More and more health researchers and practitioners are attributing diseases and ailments to high levels of stress in American society—on our jobs, at home, walking down the street, driving our cars. Some say stress may account for 85 percent *or more* of the diseases and other ailments our bodies manifest. So, what's a body to do? Take a break. Pray, meditate, take a leisurely walk in the sun, get a massage, talk, cry, take a nap, exercise, go outside and take a deep breath, breathe deeply wherever you are, take a trip, hire a babysitter for an evening, go dancing, or just don't do anything at all.

*Today I will do something nice for myself to reduce the stress level in my life.*

# DAY 15

*I have a dream.*
—MARTIN LUTHER KING, JR.

We all have dreams. The challenge is to turn dreams into reality. For those of us who are struggling with health and fitness issues, Martin Luther King, Jr., offers an excellent example of the power of persistence. He was beaten, cursed, thrown in jail, and murdered for refusing to give up. Dr. King and many other brave souls faced Jim Crow with courage and dignity. Remember what it felt like to be denied, disrespected, and rejected, simply because of your skin color? No, life in America is not perfect today, but it was blatantly worse then. Today, the war is being raged on a mental level. If your mind can be chained, then they've got you and can profit from your unhealthy habits. Persist in resisting. In a sense, it was easier for King, Malcolm X, and all the other freedom fighters to go to war because they could see their enemy clearly. For those of us who are striving for a healthy lifestyle, our enemy is not so obvious. It masquerades as ad campaigns, confusing governmental policies, public opinion, and fragmented approaches to health care.

*There are lessons to be learned*
*from the civil rights movement.*
*I will persist in resisting.*
*Knowledge is power.*

# DAY 16

*Don't quit!*

Did you think that miracles were going to happen overnight? The miracle will happen, but its manifestation will be stretched out over time. The achievement of your goals won't look like a miracle, because it will happen so slowly, naturally. But really, what is a miracle but the ability to make dreams a reality through the power of mind, intent, and persistence? You're walking on water, converting water into wine, but you're doing it inch by inch, which is the healthy way to manifest health and fitness. Taking it slowly will have long-lasting benefits. You are changing a lifetime of bad habits and laziness, so do not expect that you'll become the paragon of perfection overnight. It will take time, which you have plenty of. Just know that you are moving steadily toward your goal. Don't allow boredom, weariness, or laziness to take over. Keep on moving. Don't stop.

*I will not stop at making a miracle
happen in my body today.*

# DAY 17

*It takes an entire community to create a healthy body.*

The original African proverb, "It takes an entire village to raise a child," can be reinterpreted in light of our need for support as we pursue a healthy, fit body. Our health care must treat the whole person, not an arm here or a kneecap there. We must communicate our need for support to families and friends. Fast-food joints selling grease and sugar that proliferate in our neighborhoods should be phased out. Grocery stores must be forced to sell us only quality produce. We must fight against the overabundance of cigarette and alcohol billboards in our neighborhoods. Is it any wonder that we lead the nation in most ailments? One of the reasons why losing weight or sticking to an exercise regimen is so difficult for many of us is because we exist in unhealthy community climates. If we are serious about becoming healthy, we must become activists. We must continue to struggle against the current, while we eliminate those unhealthy influences that abound in our communities.

*I will do what I can to create a*
*healthy climate*
*in my own neighborhood.*

# DAY 18

*Eat your heart out.*

We think that holidays, special occasions, fluctuating moods, and PMS all give us license to overeat. Let's be honest with ourselves. We are a gluttonous society. We eat way beyond the point of satisfying hunger. We eat foods high in fat and low in nutritional value. Such wanton eating has led to a vast number of diseases and ailments that have sprung up in our community, and the leader is heart disease. More Black women die of heart disease than any other group. And heart disease is totally preventable. We now know that exercise and food programs that are low in fat and high in fiber and nutrients are the tickets to health and longevity. We've got the answer, so let's get busy. Cut food portions in half. Eat slowly, savoring your food. Take a breather before that second helping. You may decide you don't want it after all.

*I'm going to be good to my heart*
*today. I'll eat only*
*when I'm hungry, and I'll eat only*
*nutritionally rich foods.*

# DAY 19

*"Girl, I hate to write.*
*Why I gotta write down all this stuff?"*

A great tool of personal empowerment and self-discovery is a food-emotions journal. Most of us don't eat because we're hungry. We eat because we're tired, sad, bored, anxious, angry, lonely, depressed, even happy. We eat when we're sexually satisfied; we eat when we're not. We eat to satisfy emotional unrest, not hunger. To change from an emotional eater to one who eats to satisfy hunger, you must first bring your eating-emotional patterns to your conscious awareness. Writing down everything you eat and how you felt when you ate on a daily basis will prove an enlightening experience. Did you exercise today? Jot it down. Some experts suggest recording your weight on a weekly basis. Others say to throw the scale in the garbage and record, instead, changes in dress size. Whatever works best for you.

*I want to learn more about why I*
*eat. I will start*
*my eating-emotions journal today.*

# DAY 20

*Are you giving away your power?*

Rather than listening to our inner voices, we tend to be swayed by the desires of other people, especially our mates. Black women suffer because many of our men have accepted a body ideal that is not our own. When they tell us that we're too fat, we try to accommodate them by crash dieting or taking diet pills. When we see them (or *think* we see them) wistfully eyeing thin women, something inside of us dies. We give away our power to decide for ourselves what is best for us, and we rush right out and charge a new health club membership. We want to please and hold on to what we've got, so we try to oblige our men's fantasies (or what we *think* they are). We only end up hurting ourselves in the long run. We are seldom able to reach the goals that they, or anyone else, may have for us. Stop giving away your power. Decide for yourself your ideal body weight. If you choose to lose weight, lose it only for you.

*I will not allow anyone to make decisions about my body.*
*I will keep my power and use it to accomplish my goals.*

# DAY 21

*Food is good; food is not bad.*

Dieting is such an intense activity because so much is riding on the attainment of the perfect body. It feels as if a war is raging within us. We see the enemy as food. Food calls our names; it seduces us. We forget that food is good; food is not bad. Food gives us life. It nourishes our bodies so that we can work, play, and love efficiently and energetically. Food is not the enemy, not even high-fat food. It's how much and how frequently we eat that gets us into trouble. We have got to say *stop!* when we are no longer hungry. We can't allow ourselves to eat just because we're in a fit about something. *Food is good.* It's our miseducation about the purpose of eating that must be fixed. Let's try to see food differently today, because food is our friend. Why not go out and buy a *healthy* snack food today? Remember, eating isn't bad. What's important is *what* you eat and *how much* you eat.

*I love food, so I will not abuse food*
*or my body by overeating.*

# DAY 22

*Believe it or not, Black women have the world in the palm of their hands.*

Black women are coming from a lot of different places today. We're in school, we work, and we're housewives. No matter what we are doing, there is a common thread that weaves its way through all of our lives. We don't feel in control. There is a greeting card that depicts an African woman holding Earth in the palm of her hand. What an empowering image! The things we could do, the strides we could make if we really believed that we do indeed hold our world in the palms of our hands. It's there to shape and mold as we choose. Imagine your body as a clay figure standing right there in your open hand. The clay is soft and pliable, perfect for molding into your ideal shape. Our world—our situations, our bodies—are there to mold as we choose. We have much more power than we ever imagined.

*I see myself molding my body into
the shape I desire it to be.*

# DAY 23

*Don't get trapped by unhealthy stop-and-go cycles.*

It's a vicious cycle. We start exercising or moderating our eating in a fit of passion. We go strong for a couple of weeks, then something happens. We lose our drive. We get tired. And we quit. A month later, we start all over again. Years go by like this, and we wonder why we haven't made any changes to our bodies. You may not be conscious of the pattern of starting and stopping then starting all over again, but it's one that is controlling many of our lives. Think of your major successes in life. You weren't able to make them happen by starting and stopping. You had to press through no matter how tired you felt. To find ways to jump-start your program, ask yourself, "What turns me on?" "What makes me really happy?" Go dancing, or take a long, leisurely walk by the beach. Or try a physically challenging activity, one that you've never tried before, such as skiing, hiking, or horseback riding. Be creative.

*No more starting and stopping.*
*I'm going to take*
*a deep breath and press ahead.*

# DAY 24

*"Damn, baby, how'd you get all that in that dress?"*

Heavy women from coast to coast are busting out of society's skinny definition of how they should look. Slowly but surely they're dismantling the socially imposed rules and regulations of behavior and dress. Stores are cropping up all over the country that cater exclusively to heavy women. They're selling sexy lingerie and brightly colored dresses with space for cleavage. Vivacious women are learning that a healthy, fit lifestyle begins with self-confidence, self-love, and self-acceptance. They don't feel they have to apologize any more for anything because they're proving the old cliché to be a truth: *True beauty comes from within.* They're learning that a woman can be sick and unfit no matter what her size. The converse is also true: Heavy women can do anything skinny women can do, including dance, play volleyball, roller-skate, and make love. After all, it ain't nothing but some extra pounds.

*I'll be my own woman today.*

# DAY 25

*Get in front of the mirror, butt naked, and take an honest appraisal of your body.*

That's right, take it all off. To make it easier on you, turn this moment in front of the mirror into a real production. Turn on some sexy music, and start stripping. Have fun with yourself. Don't be embarrassed. It's your body, after all. The point is not to criticize yourself, but to honestly and lovingly look at yourself, perhaps for the first time in years, with love and acceptance. It's going to be hard. Images of Kate Moss will compete with what you see in the mirror, but resist that other woman. Know that the gorgeous creature in the mirror, rolls and all, is you. Sure, there may be parts of your body that you want to fix. Nobody's perfect. So is your stomach too big for your tastes? Do sit-ups! Is the booté going on and on and on? Walk it down! One more thing—while you're looking in the mirror, make sure you keep the lights on.

*I will look at my body today with love and acceptance.*

# DAY 26

*A strong will makes for a strong fitness program.*

You may not think you have a strong will, but you really do. Remember when you were two years old? You tried to run the house. *Mine* and *no* were your favorite words. The battle of wills fought between you and your parents drove everybody crazy. It's a difficult time, and parents usually cope by suppressing a girl's spirit, her will. Parents need to learn how to maintain their authority in the home while allowing a girl to retain her strong will. Many of us were crippled when our spirits were broken. The good thing about a break, though, is that it can be mended. Everyday you exercise, everyday you eat right, you're repairing the damage that was done to your will. Every time you say no to a cigarette or drugs or excessive alcohol or unprotected sex, you're building your will.

*My will is strong enough to help*
*me meet my health and fitness goals.*

# DAY 27

*"Why do I keep doing this to myself?"*

Does this sound like you? You weigh yourself. You've lost a couple of pounds! Like a dingdong, you go celebrate—with french fries, chocolate cake, sweet potato pie, and sundry other bits and pieces of junk food. Next day, you get on the scale, and horrors! You've gained the two pounds back! What did you expect, a miracle? Listen up: you don't have the luxury of goofing off, not until you've reached your goal. And, don't make it worse by eating more. Get back on your program right away. Put the scale in the garbage if that will help. Don't stop until you've reached your goal.

*No more acting silly.*
*I'm going to keep my promise to*
*myself and stick to my goals.*

# DAY 28

*Don't try to figure it out, 'cause*
*figuring is never gonna make you believe.*
—BIKRAM CHOUDHURY[1]

Bikram Choudhury, a teacher of Hatha Yoga to folks like Herbie Hancock and Quincy Jones, offers an intriguing mathematical formula to help us understand what happens to our bodies when we aren't consistent with our workouts. Called "the Cumulative," the formula goes something like this:

| Day 1 workout | = 5 points in the body |
|---|---|
| Day 2 workout | = 5 points in the body (subtotal: 10 points) |
| Day 3 workout | = 5 points in the body (subtotal: 15 points) |
| Grand Total | = 15 points |

Fifteen points is good. On Day 3, your body is starting to respond to exercise and believe you're really serious this time. Now let's say you miss Day 2—you lose three points. If you miss Day 3, you'll lose the last two points. When you start exercising again a few days later, you'll be stiffer, sorer, and madder than ever. The math may be crazy, but the lesson is a good one. Don't skip days. It's a drain on your motivation to have to start at zero all the time.

*Consistency is the key.*

# DAY 29

*One, two, three,* push!

If you've ever birthed a baby, you can birth a new body. Birthing a new body is just as hard, and sometimes as painful, as bringing a new life into the world. It takes strength and courage and the ability to bear pain and discomfort. As we stretch stiff bodies, tax lazy hearts, build muscle, and push past ravenous appetites to wait for hunger cues, we must learn to tolerate these new and uncomfortable feelings. When a woman is in labor, she knows she has no choice; she must have the baby. We must apply the same attitude to our pursuit of health and fitness. We have no choice. We must exercise. We must eat nutritional foods.

*I am a strong woman. I can bear the discomfort. I'll push through.*

# DAY 30

*To weigh or not to weigh?*

Some women live and die by the scale. Not a day goes by when they're not hanging their hopes and dreams on how far up the red dial moves. While there's nothing inherently wrong with weighing your body, it does foster a dependency on a mechanical device that functions outside the body's inner wisdom. We become totally dependent on a mechanical device to tell us what's going on with our bodies when we should be hearing that for ourselves. This is why most experts recommend throwing the scale in the garbage. Let's not be so drastic today. Instead, try this simple experiment: hide the scale for a week. You'll be amazed to discover the distance the scale has put between you and your body. Step back into your body and relearn its language. Don't become so dependent that you can't hear for yourself.

*I won't weigh myself today.*
*I will take the time to*
*try and hear what my body's been*
*trying to tell me.*

# DAY 31

*Could melanin be making some of us fat?*

Some people are overweight because of an addiction to carbohydrates. According to Drs. Rachael and Richard Heller in *The Carbohydrate Addict's Diet,* the carbohydrate-insulin-serotonin connection has gone ballistic. Normally, when insulin levels are high, we become hungry. After we eat, insulin levels go down, fuel is produced, and serotonin, the brain endorphin that leaves us feeling satisfied and peaceful, goes up—at least that's how it's supposed to happen. In carbohydrate addicts, insulin levels stay high, even after meals, and the nagging cravings continue on until that last gallon of ice cream. The news of this addiction may prove especially relevant to Black people in that serotonin is one of the chemical precursors to melanin, which we possess in abundance. Could it be that this same powerful blackness, this energy chemical that makes us so beautiful and suave, is also wreaking havoc with the carbohydrate-insulin-serotonin relationship? Could the reason for our collective obesity lie not in laziness, gluttony, or weak wills but in ignorance of the uniqueness of our bodies and food programs that would enhance our bodies' functioning?

*I don't know about the X factor of melanin, but I do know this: In my quest for health and fitness, I will leave no stone unturned, regardless of how strange the rock.*

# DAY 32

*We shall overcome!*

Compounding our ongoing fight against prejudice, injustice, and discrimination today is the individually waged battle against unhealthy living. With integration came the right to eat at greasy spoons. With increased leisure time came the right to watch too much TV. As more of us Black women became single parents, we have increasingly resorted to eating out, especially at fast-food restaurants. It's going to require extra work and planning, but we've got to get back into the kitchen. This is not a sexist backlash. Kitchen work is about empowerment and taking responsibility for our health. Prepare big batches of soups, greens, rice, pasta, casseroles, etc., during the weekend and freeze in clearly marked plastic bags. During the week, just defrost and reheat, creatively mix and match foods, and *voila!* good home cooking.

*I'll make the time to cook for myself.*

# DAY 33

*You've been hoodwinked. You've been bamboozled.*
—*MALCOLM X*

We should be pissed. The image industry has forced upon us impossible, undesirable standards of beauty. We are *Black* women, dammit, and while other races may flow through our veins, we are originally of African descent. We daughters of Africa have been blessed with uniquely designed bodies that have been worshiped for millennia by men the world over—except during this, our twentieth century. Our curvaceous women's bodies became fat and ugly. We're struggling with this diet thing and beating ourselves up when we don't achieve the impossible goals that have been created for us. In the meantime, the rules are changing, slowly but surely. Let's not be obsessive in an unreasonable quest for the perfect body. Perfect by whose definition? Learn to love your body type, and your love will set you free.

*I love my body just as it is.*

# DAY 34

*Forty-five percent of Black women are overweight.*
—AMERICAN DIETETIC ASSOCIATION

Forty-five percent? By whose standards? Rather than going on the defensive, let's get down to business. First of all, *we'll* decide if we're overweight. Then set a reasonable, realistic goal for your body. Second, look at creating a plan that's easy and fun enough to do for the rest of your life. Look to see how you can eliminate the sugar, salt, and fat in our dishes. Figure out how to nutritionally re-create the foods you love. Third, incorporate *fun* exercises into your new, healthy lifestyle. If aerobics gets on your nerves, turn on your favorite records and start dancing. Walk more. Play with your children. Jump rope with the girls on the block. And last but not least, move toward your goal safely and slowly. It took awhile for the pounds and inches to creep on, and it will take awhile to get them off.

*Throughout the day,
hold in your mind's eye a gorgeous
vision of a new, beautiful you.*

# DAY 35

*Ain't no mountain high enough to keep me from exercising today.*

Diana Ross had the right idea. She wasn't going to let a little thing like Mama Nature keep her from her goal. We should be just as determined to achieve our health and fitness goals. Determination is different from obsession. Obsession can lead you down a path filled with diet pills, crash diets, and images of Barbie dancing in your head. Obsession can lead to food diseases like bulimia, anorexia nervosa, and compulsive eating—all of which lead to depression. A determined woman, however, takes a balanced approach to achieving her health and fitness goals. More important, she sets reasonable, achievable goals based on her age, lifestyle, genetic makeup, and body type.

*Does my desire originate*
*from internal or external forces?*
*If internal, I know*
*I'm on the right track. If external,*
*I'll sit still in*
*order to hear my inner voice again.*

# DAY 36

*"Ooo-wee, baby."*

Artists have drawn them, photographers have photographed them. Cheeks, bottoms, derrieres, bootés, butts. Black women are famous—and envied—for their big, beautiful behinds. The image industry insists on projecting the flat behind standard, but we all know the truth: the luscious behind is the ideal. Beware of exercise advice that, if done as prescribed, would only squish lovely bootés into oblivion. The best exercises uplift and round the cheeks rather than flatten them. Squats are really good for firming and lifting the booté, as well as tightening the thighs. Walking and climbing steps are wonderful, so ignore the elevator today.

*I will not get sucked in by the hype. Love me, love my behind!*

# DAY 37

*Up you mighty women, you can accomplish what you will.*

That's exactly what Marcus Garvey would have said to us had he eavesdropped on some of our pity parties. Black woman, do you know how strong you are? You make less money than any group in the country, you suffer from more health problems than anyone else, while, in too many cases, single-handedly running a household. Let's ignore the current rash of backlash rhetoric against Black women today. Against the odds, you have managed to do what might have killed lesser women. You are the epitome of beauty, strength, and resiliency, and all the women of the world could learn from you. So now, are we going to let a little thing like getting healthy or shedding a few extra pounds get us down? Hell no. Get up off that couch. Take a walk around the block. Walk up some stairs. Give that Twinkie a second thought. Don't feel like exercising today? Why not spring-clean to your favorite songs? You can do it. You are an incredible woman.

*I got the power!*

# DAY 38

*Are you carrying the weight of the world on your body?*

Black women are famous for shouldering everyone's problems. We are the mothers, the confidantes. And when everyone else has gone to sleep, we are the ones who will wake in the middle of the night to answer a child's cries. We are the ones who personally assume responsibility for running the church, the community center, the after-school programs—even while working a full-time job. Often we respond to problems, our own and everyone else's, with food. We may not do drugs, alcohol, or cigarettes, but we sure can put away a box of cookies when no one's looking. We must learn to distance ourselves from those things we can do nothing about, and learn to lean on others if we need help coping. The myth of the Super Black Woman is no myth— we are indeed strong women. However, we run our spirits and bodies down if we do not, at least once or twice a week, act selfishly.

*Today I will put everyone on hold and put myself first.*

# DAY 39

*Ain't I a woman?*
—*SOJOURNER TRUTH*

What does it mean to be a Black woman of African descent living in America? Many of us latched onto the feminist movement of the sixties; others continue to cling to male-run religious systems. But when have we, as individuals and as a group, taken time to define our own identity? Apart from our roles as mother, wife, sister, daughter, worker, where do we fit in the universal scheme of things? Black women in America are in a state of psychological crisis. We have a twelve-in-one chance of marrying. We are, in great measure, overweight and unfit, and we lead the nation in heart disease, poverty, and a myriad of other ills. Who are we? Better yet, who should we become? We are women of strength and beauty and tenacity, who are no less deserving of love and health than any other group on the planet.

*I will not allow forces outside myself to define me. I will create the me that I want to be!*

# DAY 40

*We be cool*
—Gwendolyn Brooks

Black folks created "cool." Cool is so cool they named a cigarette after it. Black men's cool stares at you from icy, unblinking eyes that say, "I don't care." A Black woman's cool is simmering, with a hotbed of anger lurking just beneath. Her name is Sapphire. This Black woman wears a suit of armor that no one can penetrate. She goes off on folks like a firecracker and brags about it afterward. Truth is, Sapphire's shield is up because she is scared stiff of being hurt. She won't let anyone get close to her. Some of the toughest Sapphires around are overweight, using their weight as a shield. Like the Black man's machismo, Sapphire is a front for insecurity. At some point she must relinquish her simmering cool for real feelings.

*Self-love cancels out all fear. Today I will allow my natural, smiling woman to shine through.*

# DAY 41

*We must heal our watermelon shame.*

Back in the days when it was okay to make blatant, cruel fun of Black folks, we used to see images of ourselves grinning from ear to ear, eating fat, juicy slices of watermelon. This image was so cruelly used that today, when many of us see a watermelon, we go running in the opposite direction. Especially those among us who have achieved a level of economic status: "Watermelon? I eat kiwi and cantaloupe." How many of us have choked on watermelon? There's some deep collective pain there. This fruit is a symbol of this country's disrespect and mistreatment of us. It's too bad that the image-makers didn't pair us up with greasy fried chicken or coffee cake. Now that would have been a real public service. Those foods have done real damage to our hearts and thighs. And we would have been left in peace to eat our vitamin C–packed, nonfat, colon-cleansing watermelons.

*I don't give a damn, I'll make my own rules!*

# DAY 42

*CP time = Procrastination*

CP time, or "colored people's time," is Black folk slang for tardiness. We all know people who just have to be late. Our weddings and our funerals, our parties and our beauty shop appointments all start just a beat behind the clock. Of course, people on CP time come up with all kinds of excuses to be tardy, including, "My rhythms just ain't like the white man." Please. Folks who insist on arriving late to meetings have no consideration for other people's schedules, plain and simple. Now, believe it or not, CP time has a correlation to health and fitness. Are you on CP time when it comes to putting off that eating program or that exercise routine? Good news, however. There is a cure. Put this reminder all over your house: I WILL DO *IT* TODAY! "It" being your healthy eating program or your exercise routine. Put reminders on your refrigerator, doors, kitchen cabinets, toilets, and bedside table. Tape it to your wallet. No more CP time for progressive Black women!

*I'll just do it today!*

# DAY 43

*Pay attention to what your body is saying. Don't ignore persistent aches and pains.*

Believe it or not, our bodies talk to us constantly. Every growl, ache, and sneeze has meaning. It's unfortunate that we don't understand the language of our bodies. So when we have an ache, we run to the medicine cabinet. Even Western science is now beginning to admit that most of our diseases and ailments are rooted in poor nutrition and our maladjusted ways of coping with stress. Although doctors have their place—and you should always check with one if something is wrong—try to listen to what the ailment is trying to tell you. It might feel strange, but ask the ailing body part what lesson it has to share with you. Then, and this is important, trust what you hear. If a persistent cough is trying to tell you that you need to stop eating mucous-forming dairy foods, then try fasting on dairy. If chronic knee pains are begging you to lose weight, heed the warning. If high blood pressure is telling you to let go of your anger, then, honey, let it go.

*I will pay close attention to what my body's trying to tell me.*

# DAY 44

*What do you and body builders have in common?*

Carbohydrate-rich foods! If you love potatoes, sweets, spaghetti, rice, and bread, then you share a dependence on a common food type. While body builders scientifically load up on certain carbs for energy and *to deliberately gain weight,* we tend to use foods like pasta, rice, and potatoes (loaded with fat) to help us stretch meals and to leave us feeling full. Current diet industry wisdom places the blame for heaviness squarely on fats, but for many of us, the problem may be caused by a biochemical disorder called "carbohydrate addiction," according to Drs. Rachael and Richard Heller of the Mount Sinai School of Medicine in New York.[2]

The basis for the addiction is a chemical ménage à trois gone bad among carbohydrates, insulin, and serotonin. Not every overweight person is addicted, nor is every addicted person overweight. However, this disorder may prove an important clue in the journey to health and fitness for many Black women. The Hellers cite years of research, interesting case studies, and a self-test in their best-selling book, *The Carbohydrate Addict's Diet.* Your homework assignment: study your body and read the book

*My body is the laboratory, and my
will and intelligence are the keys to
unlocking the mysteries of health
for my body.*

# DAY 45

*Don't forget the ivories.*

Unless the dentist is cute and single, probably our least favorite activity in the world is having our teeth examined. Something about the drilling so close to our brains. As women, however, we can't afford to be lax about the ivories that CHEW OUR FOOD! Our teeth are particularly sensitive to all the hormonal changes we experience during menstruation, pregnancy, and menopause; and because Western doctors tend to treat pieces of us rather than all of us, we forget that all of our cells, organs, and systems are interconnected and interdependent. Teeth feel a bit shaky? To make sure nothing's wrong, by all means have your teeth checked. Get annual cleanings (or more frequently if your dentist says so). Go easy on sugar-loaded foods. Some of the latest research says that a stick of sugarless gum a day will keep the dentist away. Or try massaging your teeth and gums with a wooden licorice stick (you can buy these at most health food stores). Our African ancestors swore by them.

*I don't want raggedy teeth. I'm*
*calling my dentist today.*

# DAY 46

*Don't quit!*

When you don't feel motivated, and nothing—no affirmations, no visualizations, nothing—can get you exercising, that's when you need to close your eyes and just
do it anyway. Don't think about how hard it is to take
that extra mile. Just do it. Think instead of the new
wardrobe you're going to buy once you've met your
goals. Think of sex, anything to get you through. The
hardest times, if you master them, can push you to
higher levels of health and fitness. So now is not the time
to stop. Do something different. Sing while you work
out. Change your walking route. Buy pretty new sweats.

*I'm not going to stop. I'm going to
keep on keeping on. I can do this.*

# DAY 47

*If you're overwhelmed by the bigness of your health goal, break it down into small, manageable pieces.*

Women who choose weight loss over weight maintenance can feel overwhelmed by the numbers—the number of pounds you want to lose, the amount of time it's going to take to get there, the number of calories and fat grams you're allowed per day—it's enough to make you scream for mercy. What's needed is some good ole Black woman ingenuity. Reframe in your mind the parameters of your goal. Think of smaller, more manageable short-term goals. Achievement of these smaller pieces will give you that feeling of accomplishment you so desperately need along the way. So instead of saying, "I want to lose one hundred pounds," give yourself a weight loss goal of ten pounds. Reward yourself when you succeed. Most of weight loss is a psyche job. It's a process of mental toughening and imagination work. Olympic athletes often attribute their success not to physical ability, but the strenuous mental work they did prior to competition.

*I will rethink my narrow definitions of success.*

# DAY 48

*Eat your roughage.*
—*Your Mama*

The industry calls it fiber today, but let's call it what our mamas called it—roughage, broom food that sweeps through and cleans out the intestines and colons. The health of your body's elimination system is totally dependent on a diet with lots of roughage. And a colon impacted with years' worth of toxins may account for a whole host of cancers and other diseases. Vegetables, of course, are great. Just don't overcook them. Steaming and stir-frying is best. Oatmeal with a dash of salt, fresh raspberries or strawberries, and brown sugar first thing in the morning will have you feeling good and cleaned out by the end of the day. Beans are also good; just soak and cook them well to eliminate gas. Beans, veggies, and oats are also naturally low in fat and high in nutrients. A diet rich in roughage eliminates the need for laxatives.

*It's a dirty business, but somebody's got to do it!*

# DAY 49

*Once upon a time . . .*

. . . there was a Black woman named Carrie. She never had a weight problem until her late teens, when she hooked up with a man who liked to beat her up. Carrie finally managed to get out of the abusive relationship, but not before some scars were seared into her soul. An attractive woman, Carrie thought that the only way to protect herself from men was to grow. So she did. She ate herself into oblivion, all the while dieting and fretting about her weight. Fortunately, this story has a happy ending. Through the process of therapy and inner work, Carrie began to understand her unconscious reasons for her obesity. Slowly but surely, she embarked on a program of exercise and sensible eating. At thirty-four, Carrie is now the same weight she was in her late teens. And if any man thinks about laying a hand on her, she's got a mean right hook for them. The moral of the story is, if Carrie can do it, you can too.

Why *did I allow my body to get into this condition?*

# DAY 50

*Water therapy is the prescription for stress, aches, and pains.*

Wouldn't it be nice to take a flight to the nearest mineral bath? Our lives are so hectic, we need regular $H_2O$ breaks to soothe frayed nerves. And as we get older, the aches and pains seem to become more numerous. The next best thing to getting away from it all is stepping into your own tub in the privacy of your own bathroom. To prepare, clean up the bathroom, bring in some flowers or plants, hang a couple of pictures with tranquil scenes on the wall. Keep the colors in your bathroom muted and subdued, to give it a luxurious feeling. You also might consider investing in a whirlpool attachment for the tub. There's nothing better than warm water vigorously massaging tired, achy muscles. Now, light a couple of candles, turn on the jazz, throw in a handful or two of your favorite scented bath salts, and *soak*. Time out. Take a bath after a long, hard day at work or after playing with the kids, or after a strenuous workout. Your body will thank you.

*I'm going to put on my headphones, tune out the world, and soak.*

# DAY 51

*"Oh, no, broccoli again?"*

We know we should be eating grains, legumes, fruits, and vegetables. So why do we continue to binge on potato chips and pie? "I can't stand rabbit food." "Beets? Yech." To quote your mama, "Tough!" The truth is, we need certain foods because of their high nutritional content. The good news is that you can change your taste buds. Many of our taste preferences were acquired, which means we can reprogram our taste buds to enjoy nutritionally rich foods—*even* broccoli. There are a million and one cookbooks on the market. Experiment. It's amazing what low-fat spinach dip can do for raw carrots. Just remember, when cooking veggies, don't overcook—steaming and stir-frying are best. Lay off the salt pork and try herbs like thyme and rosemary. Garlic, of course, is a great, healthy way to perk up vegetables.

*I use the powers of intention, determination, and creativity to reprogram my misbehaving taste buds.*

# DAY 52

*"Carrot juice? Naw, girl, I don't think so."*

Feeling tired? Irritable? Just never seem to have enough energy to get through the day? Getting colds and the flu a lot? If you answered yes to most, if not all, of the above, your immune system is on the blitz or, as our mamas used to say, "Girl, you're run-down." Juicing has, in recent years, become a popular and powerful self-help method of boosting tired, run-down bodies back into health. A juicer extracts the juice from most available parts of the fruit or vegetable, leaving only the seeds and skin behind. Unlike cooking, which removes many of a food's nutrients, juicing leaves all nutrients intact. Some hard-core health nuts drink stuff like carrot and garlic juice, but if you're not so adventurous, try fruit juices first. Or try blending veggies with fruit. Carrots and apples make a good mix. A dash of fresh ginger will really perk up the taste. Store-bought juices can't begin to compare in taste, freshness, and nutritional content to the juices you can make at home with a minimal investment of time and money. Price a juicer today. There's bound to be one in your price range.

*A fresh juice a day will make the doctor stay away.*

# DAY 53

*Who is your role model?*

Rosa Parks, Ida B. Wells, Mary McCloud Bethune, Bessie Coleman, Mahalia Jackson, Fannie Lou Hamer, Harriet Tubman, Sojourner Truth, Lena Horne—just to name a few. Why are they role models? Because they lost five pounds and kept it off for ten years? No! They did great things for their people. Their lives had meaning and purpose. When you are working at something you love, being a couple of pounds overweight loses its earth-shattering significance. Ida B. Wells was a fearless journalist who traveled the South, documenting the lynchings of Black men. Rosa "I'm Tired" Parks virtually started the civil rights movement with her one act of defiance. Harriet Tubman took slaves to freedom, some of them kicking and screaming all the way. We love our Black heroines not for their size, but for their courage and contributions to the elevation of our race.

*I've got this dieting business in perspective now.*

# DAY 54

*Are you eating to cope?*

OK, you know you need to confront the situation, but you just can't seem to get the energy, or courage, to face it. Instead, you push it down deep with food. Like Carter G. Woodson said, we negroes been real miseducated. How did we ever come to believe that eating a food, especially a sweet or a salty, fatty food, would make a problem disappear? There is no logic there, and yet we continue to eat to push down uncomfortable emotions. So many of us have been coping with unresolved problems by eating for so long that we eat automatically now. We don't even think about it. Boss is pissing you off, grab a cookie. Bored, eat potato chips. Mad at mate, eat ice cream. First plan of attack is to realize what you're doing. Remember our food-emotions journal? If you've been diligent, you should start seeing some interesting patterns emerging.

 *I'm going to deal with that problem today, and I won't have a cookie before, during, or after.*

# DAY 55

*You're only as sick as your secrets.*

What are you hiding from yourself? It's bad enough that we wear masks to cover our true selves from friends and strangers, but when we wear the masks to hide from ourselves, then we've got a problem. We're in danger of forgetting who we really are, and when we forget who we are, we forget the reasons why we allowed our bodies to become unfit and unhealthy in the first place. We create myths to replace the buried truth—Mama did it, Daddy did it, if only I was given more love as a child, we say. Most of us haven't a clue about our subconscious motivations. You owe it to yourself to get to the root of your issues. Peel away the masks of shame, anger, pain, and blame, and look deeply within. Seek out the truth of your unhealthy habits so that you will not be destined to repeat them throughout your days. You might be amazed to discover that you're not as bad as you thought; in fact, you're quite adorable, faults and all.

*My mask is removed.*
*I want to see the truth of*
*me, no matter how scary.*

# DAY 56

*What is a fat?*

Basically, there are three types of fat: saturated, monounsaturated, and polyunsaturated. Saturated fat is bad
for the heart and cholesterol levels. Saturated fats are
found in dairy products, especially cheeses and butter,
as well as red meat. Monounsaturated (olive oil, nuts)
and polyunsaturated (vegetable oils) fats can have a positive effect in lowering cholesterol levels. However,
polyunsaturated fats can have a negative effect on the
immune system. How much fat should you include in
your daily food program? Some experts say obese
women should keep fat to around 10 percent of calories—others say 20 to 30 percent. Talk with your doctor about it. In addition, read packaging labels. "Lite"
and "lean" do not necessarily mean low fat. Learn how
to cut the fat out of your favorite soul food dishes. All
you'll be giving up are the unwanted pounds and health
problems.

*I will use the formula that
Susan Powter made famous:
Number of fat grams × 9 = X
X ÷ total calories = X % of fat per
serving.*

# DAY 57

*"Girl, when I walk, it's like making a fire!"*

Think that chairs are only made for sitting? What a waste of use! Chairs are great for exercising your inner thighs. Simply sit on the floor, wrap your feet securely around the legs and squeeze tight. Hold for 20 seconds, then release. Repeat the sequence 10 times, and in a few weeks your inner thighs will be jiggle-free. Isometric exercises reduce the risk of injury, and they work deeply into the muscles. Now stand up and hold the chair for balance. Do 30 leg kicks—10 to the front, 10 to the side, 10 to the back. Repeat on the other side. Say, when was the last time you wore a miniskirt?

*My chair is no longer just a piece of furniture. It has been transformed!*

# DAY 58

*What are we thinking?*

Do you believe that there is such a thing as race or group consciousness? The 1990 census counted approximately 16 million Black women in this country. That's 16 million Black women thinking a zillion thoughts every day. Many of those thoughts we share, like, "I'm so fat," "All men are dogs," "I need me a man," "I'm so tired," and "She's so thin, I can't stand her." Much of what we are thinking and feeling as a group is negative and has polluted the atmosphere in our communities. Now imagine a new group mind, one that values self-love, self-confidence, and self-acceptance above all else, one that places educational and behavioral emphasis on creating and maintaining healthy lifestyles. All it takes is a new attitude, and we could obliterate in an eye blink the diseases and ailments that plague us as a group.

*My contribution to the Black woman group mind is important. I will make every effort to think and behave in ways that promote self-love and health.*

# DAY 59

*Let's look to the elder beauties for guidance and
inspiration.*

We all know at least one elder beauty. She's a woman
of beauty, class, and sophistication. Her manners are im-
peccable, and she's won the hard-earned right to be
honest and forthright. But even when she's telling
you off, you feel as if you've been blessed by someone
with wisdom. Her hair is often gray, with a sharp, well-
maintained cut. Her clothes refuse to date her. She can
wear a miniskirt or a leather suit without appearing as
if she's dressing too young for her age. She always looks
good, and she makes you think, "I want to be just like
her when I grow up." Elder beauties are great role models for those of us struggling with issues like self-love,
self-confidence, and self-acceptance. Talk to them. Get
them to share their health and beauty secrets with you.
Beg an elder beauty to adopt you. You'll come to appreciate the decades they've dedicated to making their
lives a work of art. Years of struggle and determination
have brought them to this place of peace.

*My senior years don't fill me with
dread anymore.
Elder beauties in my community
are showing me the way.*

# DAY 60

*Are you starved for affection?*

We all need it bad. We need to be touched, hugged, caressed. Babies will die if they're not touched. We adults, on the other hand, don't have sense enough to die. We go crazy. Instead of reaching out and getting our sugar, we feed our starving needs with food. What sense does that make? Our miseducation has led us to believe that this is a rational solution to an unbearable problem, but it is not, and we go nuts! Women, go out and get your hugs today, and no duck hugs with butts sticking out allowed! Hug deeply and warmly, as if your life depended on holding the person. Be lusty. Hug your children. They love it and need it too. Hug your man. You know he wants it. Hug your sisterfriends. Meet somebody just for the purpose of hugging him. Hug your mama, hug your daddy. Hug an old person. Folks may think you've gone off the deep end, but after their initial shock wears off, they'll begin to like it. Finally, before you go to bed, give yourself a massive hug.

*So many hugs, so little time!*

# DAY 61

*"Girl, I gets down on the dance floor."*

Most Black folks love to dance. Dancing is one of the most fun ways to stay in shape. Turn on the box, play your favorite music, and get to stepping. Have your kids teach you the latest dance steps. Teach them some of your old ones. For upper body strength and development, try cabbage patching. As you're rotating your arms around and around (like you're stirring a thick batter in a huge bowl), make sure your upper body is kept somewhat rigid for maximum effectiveness. Remember the penguin? Kick your legs out to each side and to the beat. That dance is great for overall toning of the legs, especially the thighs. When was the last time you went out for an evening of fun and dance? Steppers sets[3] and house parties provide great opportunities to have some fun exercise as well as meet new men. Or if you have a man, drag him out of the house for a dancing night out on the town. Just take it easy on the alcohol, which is loaded with calories.

*I'm going to get out my red dancing shoes today, and cut up a serious rug!*

# DAY 62

*Be a pro-health role model for your children.*

It's a sad truth, but Bebe's kids are getting big and fat as they sit in front of the TV day in and day out, mimicking *your* behavior. If they see you active and not TV-addicted, then they will be active. Black folks watch more TV than any other racial group in the country. What's with this marathon TV watching with our people? Imagine the things we could be doing if we weren't watching TV. We could be learning new skills, developing relationships with our children, building financial empires, cleaning up our neighborhoods, and creating fit, healthy bodies. Unless you're working out with one of the many exercise shows, TV is a big waste of time. And our children are getting fatter and fatter. Turn off the TV. After dinner, take a walk together. Read books together. Talk to each other.

*I owe it to my children to be fit and healthy. My children deserve a healthy mother.*

# DAY 63

*Cravings are windows of spiritual opportunity.*

Black folks are some of the most spiritual people in the world, but how often do we remember to draw from that rich wellspring within the deepest parts of our souls when cravings overwhelm us? We tend to look to outside sources for strength. We buy books and diet club memberships. We ask our mates silly questions like, "Am I fat?" Probably the most self-destructive thing we do when stressed out. When you try to erase uncomfortable feelings with food, you miss the opportunity to learn from the cravings, many of which are tied to the emotions, usually negative ones. The only way to get control of your cravings is to feel them completely. Take a walk. Do some deep breathing. Talk positively to yourself. After a while, the feeling will go away. And you will have learned something about yourself.

*When a strong craving hits, I will close my eyes and listen to what it is trying to tell me.*

# DAY 64

*What's cellulite got to do with it?*

Tina Turner has some of the most beautiful legs on the planet, and why shouldn't she? She's dancing all the time! Most of us have not made a career of dancing. Or exercising. Most of us are sitting behind a desk all day and on the couch all night watching TV. Even if we've incorporated a half-hour or so of exercise into our days, we're probably not going to have the super-incredible bodies that have been held up as a standard by the media—unless we were so blessed by nature. We need to rethink this issue of cellulite. It can be minimized by exercise and eating fresh, healthy, nonfat foods, but in the final analysis, what does cellulite have to do with having a happy life? Nothing! Once again, we've been bamboozled by a money-grubbing diet industry looking for any cheap way to make a buck. We've bought into a nonissue. Cellulite is not life-threatening in any way, shape, or form.

*My beautiful thighs are perfect.*
*They keep me standing tall.*

# DAY 65

*A big appetite is a sure sign of a lusty woman.*

Our society does not approve of women with big appetites—in anything. Women with small appetites are considered feminine and dainty; women with huge appetites are masculine, threatening, and dangerous. We must pretend to want only one helping of food. Anything more brings down the judgmental glares of others. Traces of social repression still exist in most aspects of our lives and we often use food to push down big life appetites that are not socially acceptable. What are our appetites telling us? Seek to unveil the secret that lies hidden in your big appetite by refusing to feed it. Usually, when the appetite hits, our first inclination is to calm it down. Don't do that today. Listen to your emotions and your body as they scream their displeasure. Unsatisfied appetites cause great discomfort, but also contain golden nuggets of information.

*My appetite for life is big and juicy. I'm going to find out just what I've been missing.*

# DAY 66

*Heavy Black Woman = Mammy = Nurturer?*

The archetype of the heavy Black woman is deeply embedded in the American psyche. Butterfly McQueen and the old Aunt Jemima epitomize the American ideal of Black womanhood. Hollywood and Corporate America have given her a one-dimensional role of servant-nurturer. Everyone lies comforted in her big, meaty arms. This mammy has no other purpose in life but to attend to other people's dreams. She has no dreams or goals, and even today, allusions to mammy creep up in the conversation of white America. How does this persistent image of Black womanhood affect us today? Others may feel comfortable with us when we are big, but what happens to relationships when we lose weight? On an "Oprah" show about this very issue, many women expressed their dismay at Oprah's weight loss. Her wealth did not bother them; her weight loss did. The lessons we learn from Oprah's weight loss? You can't please everybody, so only aim to please yourself. It's going to take a lot to dismantle the mammy-as-nurturer archetype.

*I ain't nobody's mammy! I am a beautiful*
*Black woman no matter what my size.*

# DAY 67

*Eat all your food. There's people starving in India.*
—*YOUR MAMA*

Since we've grown up, many of us have rebelled against the notion that what's on our plates has something to do with the empty stomachs of people half a world away. As we're eating to fill emotional needs, or eating way past the point of hunger, let's face it, we don't want to think of starving people. It's hard to reconcile excessive, unnecessary eating to the fact that there are indeed starving people in the world. Maybe Mama was wrong. How can *excessive* eating be helpful when other people are starving?

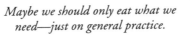

*Maybe we should only eat what we need—just on general practice.*

# DAY 68

*The quest for health and fitness is a religious one.*

The most successful religions in the world use rituals to create an aura of mystery. The best rituals make beliefs tangible and real through the involvement of our bodies—our senses, speech, etc. Ritual strengthens our faith and plunges us deeper into the mysteries of our belief. It is the peculiarity of Western society that our lives are compartmentalized; ritual is meant for the church service, not everyday living. Because of the lack of ritual on a day-to-day basis, our lives feel mundane and less than holy. Exercising is not the transcendent experience it should be; it is often tedious and boring. It's time that we incorporate rituals in our efforts. Pray for strength before exercising, and, like the Muslims, pray with your entire body. Play inspirational music, like Gospel, to get your body excited and moving. Stretch high to heaven in yoga asanas (postures) as you seek help. The Catholics use incense to create mood and atmosphere. Experiment. And before you take a bite, give thanks and affirm the nourishment the food provides.

*I will infuse my health and fitness activites with ritual.*

# DAY 69

*Confession is good for the soul.*

Can we talk? Some of our deepest, darkest secrets are as plain as the weight on our bodies. Unhappiness with men is an important source of secrets, but come on, we can't blame everything on them. How about our secret fears, failures, and shames? Deep down, every woman carries a secret, and some of us carry it on our bodies. Black women have additional issues of skin color and hair length. During religious services, we kiss, we smile, we hug each other, all the while pretending that we're just fine. "I'm blessed," we smile bravely. But we're not just fine if we're sick or obese, and we need to stop faking. We need to get real. Unburden yourself and confess your secrets—not to just any old body, but to someone you trust. If there's no one, talk it out with a professional. Shame-based secrets are like weights on the body that fester and grow into illnesses and diseases.

*It's time I resolved my issues.*
*I'm tired of carrying them around*
*on my body.*

# DAY 70

*Massage stress off your body.*

There ain't nothing like a good massage for whatever ails you. Boss getting on your last nerves? Get a massage. Strenuous workout? Get a massage! Our skin, joints, and muscles all crave the deep manipulation of a good massage. There are many different types of massage to deal with a variety of bodily conditions. Some of the best stress-busting massages occur during sex. Professional masseuses are also well worth the investment. If you can't afford a professional, buy a foot massager or a hand-held model for shoulder and neck areas. A friend kneading your neck and shoulder muscles can also be quite relaxing. Always have fragrant lotions or oils available. For example, eucalyptus leaves soaked in almond oil makes an inexpensive massage oil.

*Even if I've got to do it myself,*
*I'm going to get my muscles*
*massaged.*

# DAY 71

*A pretzel by any other name is still an asana.*

If ever there was a miracle exercise it's yoga. Said to have originated in ancient Egypt, yoga is a wonderful mind-body discipline. It combines deep levels of concentration with specialized breathing and scientific exercises designed to stretch, strengthen, and heal the body inside and out. Yoga has been adapted especially for the physically challenged, the obese, women, and the elderly. After only a short time of practice, you'll begin to feel remarkable changes in your body. Achy joints feel better, stomach irritations are soothed, and blood pressure often stabilizes. Yoga is a wonderful remedy for many PMS symptoms; for example, asanas like "the Cobra" relieve back pain. Teachers are quick to point out that yoga will not cure ailments, and if you don't practice the asanas, the old aches and pains will surely return. There are many books and tapes on the market, but beginners should practice under the watchful eye of an experienced master. Look in the phone book, or ask around for recommendations. You can try one class for very little money. If you like it, sign up for the program.

*Yoga sounds like an interesting change of pace. I think I'll give it a try.*

# DAY 72

*Say "no!" to breast cancer.*

Obesity is not the worse thing that comes with a high-fat, low-movement lifestyle. Researchers are now beginning to link certain forms of breast cancer to obesity. In particular, diets high in animal fats (vs. vegetable fats) are being viewed as the culprits. That means the typical Black diet. Black women are famous for their ability to throw down in the kitchen, but the foods that we are famous for are precisely what might be killing us. We season collards with salt pork. Have you ever seen a skinny pig? Anything so saturated with salt can't be good for you. And what about our favorite—sweet potato pie? Sweet potatoes are great, it's the butter and sugar that causes so many problems. Macaroni and cheese? Macaroni is a good, high-carbohydrate food, but the cheese and the butter are really bad fats. The good news is that many breast cancers may be preventable. Don't give up soul food—just redesign it. We have no choice in this. It's a matter of life and death.

*I will reduce the fat in my diet to keep myself fit and healthy.*

# DAY 73

*"Girl, I feel sick. I think I ate too much."*

You know you've done it too. Your eyes and appetite
are bigger than your stomach, and you feel as if you simply cannot resist gorging yourself. You start out with
good intentions, but the meal gets to tasting so good,
and satisfies (temporarily) so many needs, that you eat
fast to keep from thinking about how much you are eating. You're on automatic. You're no longer tasting anything. Then suddenly, it hits you. You're as sick as a dog.
All you can do now is lie down, be quiet, and wait for
the discomfort to pass. Some women make themselves
throw up (bulimia only makes a bad situation worse).
We've got to learn to *stop eating when we're no longer
hungry.* Drink two or three glasses of water before your
meal. Chew your food at least twenty times. Take
smaller bites. Give your stomach time to tell you when
it's full.

*From now on,*
*I'll stop eating when I'm satisfied.*

# DAY 74

*Imagine yourself ten years into the future.*

What do you look like? Have you made any progress in your health and fitness program, or are you still talking about starting your diet on Monday? Now imagine that you can actually talk to this older version of yourself, only make her body 20 pounds heavier. Ask her what she would have done differently ten years ago (your age today). Make this exercise real to you. An older you will have much to say about procrastination, taking risks, discipline, and dreaming big. She'll be able to see how the many binges and sedentary nights in front of the TV have accumulated over time. Now imagine yourself ten years older, but this time with the body you've always wanted. Ask her to advise you on how to proceed. See this woman clearly, and heed her wise words. Let her take you by the hand and lead you to the promised land.

*Ten years is just around the corner.
I have a lot of talking to do with
myself.*

# DAY 75

*Don't quit!*

Sometimes it's all you can do to get yourself out of bed, much less exercise. The danger in quitting now, though, is that you'll lose a lot of the progress you've made so far. (Remember the Cumulative?) You've worked so hard, it would be a shame to gain back a pound or two, or lose the muscle tone that's finally beginning to take shape. You'll also lose momentum, for if you allow yourself to quit today, what's to stop you from goofing off tomorrow or the next day? It's just not worth it. If, however, you are really exhausted, it would be counterproductive to try to run at your usual level of intensity. An alternative is to walk at a leisurely pace. The point is to keep moving. Tomorrow you can work your way back up to speed. And hey, if you *really* want that damn ice-cream cone, have it! Just work it off tomorrow.

*I'm not going to stop. My goal is like a light at the end of the tunnel.*

# DAY 76

*"Raw vegetables? Where's the salt pork?"*

Nutritionists tell us that munching on raw veggies is a great way to curb a raging appetite. And of course, raw vegetables pack a much more powerful nutritional punch than when cooked. As potent as they are, however, they can be a bit hard to take. Raw carrots and celery sticks just don't compare to a slice of chocolate cake. So what's called for is some old-fashioned creativity. Low-fat salsas and dips can surely make raw veggies much more palatable. Raw celery sticks stuffed with low-fat cream cheese can actually rival a good butter cookie. Throw raw veggies into a tossed salad and top with low-fat dressing. You'll be amazed at how satisfying that can be. Another approach is to make raw veggie sandwiches. Lettuce, spinach, tomatoes, cucumbers, sprouts, and shredded carrots, with low-fat mayonnaise and mustard, sandwiched in a toasted plain bagel or whole grain bread with a *thin* slice of cheese is heaven. A nice bonus to be earned from eating raw vegetables is the energy you'll gain.

*I will call on all my powers of creativity
to make raw vegetables a
delicious treat.*

# DAY 77

*Pucker up!*

Just looking at a lemon can make your cheeks curdle, but Sister, are they great for you. We love to squirt lemon in our water, teas, and over salad and fish. There's nothing as refreshing as fresh, homemade lemonade on a hot summer day. Lemons are high in vitamin C, which makes them an essential food in our efforts to build the immune system. Their citric acid content is high, so dilute with water and drink in moderation. Lemons are great for cleaning out the small intestine. Lemons may even help increase energy levels and enhance metabolic balance.[4]

*Lemons make my health sweet, not sour.*

# DAY 78

*"Girl, it's hard being a woman."*

How you proceed through the biological milestones in your life has much to do with the quality of your character. Those milestones give your life shape and depth. The growth of breasts, menstruation, childbearing, and menopause are important moments that affect how we view the world and how others view us. Furthermore, each stage brings its own set of challenges to health and fitness. We all know about the cramps, bloating, and irritability that's often associated with PMS. Our bodies retain fat by design as we bear children. More hormonal changes and psychological challenges accompany menopause. Enter Western society and its decidedly antinature, antiwoman, anti-African approach to life. Society has created a very narrow picture of womanhood and many of the elements run contrary to our life stages. This may only aggravate the state of our health as we try to fit the mold. As we redefine Black womanhood for ourselves, let's also reinterpret the natural stages of a woman's life as positive, each one full of growth potential rather than something to be dreaded.

*I honor each stage of my life as a
Black woman.*

# DAY 79

*"Girl, I just can't take it."*

When a catastrophe happens in your life, how do you handle it? What's your style of coping? The death of a loved one, the breakup of a relationship, illness, accidents, and job loss can affect our appetites in different ways. Some of us binge the long, lonely nights away, while for others, the mere sight of food brings on waves of nausea. How we respond to major stress is a personal issue; there's no right or wrong way. What is important, though, is that we take responsibility for our healing. We can't allow ourselves to stay submerged in our grief, because the longer we do so, the more we put our health at risk. Eventually we must take our place in the flow of life, and that might mean getting help. There's a stigma attached to therapy in our community, but we've got to want our healing so badly it matters not what others say.

*My spiritual, physical, and
emotional help is
what matters now. I will do
whatever it takes
to feel whole again.*

# DAY 80

*There's gold at the end of the rainbow.*

The rainbow is a powerful visual metaphor for our journey to emotional health and physical fitness. Beginning our program and overcoming all sorts of internal and external resistance is much like climbing up the hill to the rainbow. Climbing upward represents the struggle against ourselves—our lack of confidence—and the slow progress toward our goals. But as we reach the peak of the hill, we grow stronger. We're nurtured by the warm rays of the sun. The trek down is as easy as riding a bike downhill. We're much more confident. We're on a roll. We've built positive momentum, and we're finally seeing progress. Of course, the pot of gold at the end of the rainbow is the attainment of our goals, and once we're on flat land we move into a maintenance mode. The many colors of the rainbow symbolize the beauty and power of our spirit, which is that part of us that gives us the strength and the vision.

*I'm a rainbow spirit, powerful in my ability to achieve my goals.*

# DAY 81

*Don't panic!*

As stressful as life in America can be, it's a wonder that we're all *not* in a constant state of panic. We all feel anxious at times, but women who are prone to clinical attacks of anxiety can feel totally out of control *all* of the time. Apart from the overwhelming feeling of panic, sufferers manifest such symptoms as racing hearts, cramping, chest pain, dizziness, and nausea. More and more of us are resorting to antidepressants, like Prozac and Xanax, but you'll never heal that way. Drugs are only a temporary solution to a problem that may go soul deep. To truly heal, you must get to the root of the trouble. A therapist can help you navigate the often frightening avenues of memory, as well as teach you calming techniques.

*I will try to be calm and worry-free
for one day,
then one week, then one month.
My goal is to be
calm and worry-free the rest of
my days.*

# DAY 82

*De knee bone's connected to de thigh bone, now hear de word of de Lord.*
—NEGRO SPIRITUAL

Our skeleton is the system that gives our body shape and structure. As we women get older, we must address our increased need for calcium. The older we get, the higher the risk of bone thinning, or osteoporosis. In fact, more than half of women over the age of forty-five have some form of the bone disease. In advanced stages, bones become brittle and are more susceptible to breaking. Women walk over stooped, and suffer a lot of pain. Fortunately, we can prevent it. To build density in the bones, we must boost our daily calcium intake and—surprise!—exercise. Nutritionists encourage us to drink at least three glasses of non- or low-fat milk a day. Many Black women can't stand the watery taste of skim milk; others are lactose intolerant. Don't despair! Calcium can be found in a favorite soul food dish of ours—collard greens. In addition, a study out of London found calcium supplements to be effective in enhancing bone density. Isn't it nice to know that here's yet another disease that can be prevented through nutrition and exercise?

*My bones are precious to me. I need them, and I'm going to take good care of them.*

# DAY 83

*Violence is a public health issue.*
—Centers for Disease Control

There's been a lot of talk lately about our young Black people and their strange otherworldly ways. Violence among youth has risen to an all-time high. In fact, the leading killer of young Black men is not disease but homicide. In addition to high teen pregnancy rates, many young females are also resorting to violence and gang participation. The Centers for Disease Control in Atlanta call violence a public health problem, and if you accept this view, then our community is over-whelmed with sickness. Where do these kids get these sick behaviors? you may ask. Let's answer that question with some more questions. How do *you* resolve conflict? Do *you* engage in risky sexual activity? Do *you* drink and smoke? Are *you* obese? The point is, our children learn by example. They're not aliens. They're simply acting out behaviors they've learned from us.

*First I change the woman in the mirror, then I change the world.*

# DAY 84

*Black folks speak the language of food.*

"Give me some sugar." "Come here, sweetie pie, honey bunch." "The blacker the berry the sweeter the juice." We even have nicknames like "Puddin'." From the way we talk, you can tell we love to eat. Some of our best times come from eating great meals. We associate food preparation with love. Leaving food on the plate is an insult to a Black cook. Some Black women have created their identities around their ability to nourish loved ones. Also, feasts are a big part of our culture. Food represents prosperity and the promise of better times to come. We celebrate with food, and we mourn with food. No other race of people eat more at a wake than we do. The problem with all this focusing on food is that we feast on high-fat food while our community is plagued by diet-related diseases and ailments. Also, with some women, our love of food becomes an obsession. Rather than dealing with problems, we eat them into hiding. There's nothing inherently wrong with using food to celebrate special occasions. It's an important part of our culture. Just remember two things: (1) Keep eating in perspective—it's not who we are, it's one of the things we do to nourish and fuel our bodies. (2) Please, convert to low-fat cooking, for the health of yourself and your loved ones.

*Vive la low-fat food!*

# DAY 85

*Detox for the sake of your health.*

If ever there was a risk to health and sanity, an addiction to drugs and alcohol is it. The media sensationalizes the plight of those Black women who are addicted to crack-cocaine or other drugs, which casts a pall over all of us. Is the media blowing the rate of addiction among Black females out of proportion, or are we all paragons of virtue? The truth probably lies somewhere in the middle of these two extremes. While most of us are probably not junkies, many of us, in the loneliness of a long, empty night or while socializing with friends, probably do have an occasional one too many. Just be careful. Even social drinking can lead to addiction, and the impact of alcohol and drugs on personal finances is enormous. The answer is to find other positive outlets to express joy and abandon, spiritual connection, and emotional healing.

*Addiction is just not worth it.*
*I am clean, healthy,*
*and happy. I will explore*
*alternative ways to get a*
*natural high.*

# DAY 86

*Will builder: Give celibacy a try.*

The only way to progress is to exercise the faculty of will. We all are born with it. (Just watch any two-year-old in action.) Giving celibacy a try is one way to build the will. Single women, abstain from sex until Mr. Wonderful comes along. If you're in a monogamous, committed relationship (like marriage), talk it over with your partner and explain to him what you're trying to do. If he's adamantly opposed to the idea, then save it for another time. But if he's willing to give it a try, go without sex for no longer than a week or two. Use the time in prayer and meditation. Get to know yourself again. Channel excess sexual energy into creative projects and workouts. And when you start *doing it* again, the loving will be that much sweeter.

*A short-term vacation from sex
refreshes my mind and body.*

# DAY 87

*There's a new dance in town, and it's called the
Running Woman.*

Ever heard of a crazy dance called the Running Man?
Well, now there's the Running Woman, and it's a great
aerobic workout. We Black women do the Running
Woman every day of our lives. We run to the store. We
run to clean the snot out of the kid's nose. We run to
the cleaners. We run the kids to school. We run to
work. Hey, Running Woman, it's time to slow down.
Put everybody and everything on hold. Don't run anywhere. Just sit still for a minute.

*I'm going to calm down.
Everybody can wait.*

# DAY 88

*Exercise is big business.*

How many of us have bought a piece of exercise equipment, and even used it a couple of times, only to relinquish it to a corner in the basement as a plant hanger? Exercise equipment ain't cheap, but we spend the money anyway because of the strong sales pitch promising slender bodies. Exercise equipment can work, but only if you use it consistently. If you must buy one, keep the following pointers in mind: (1) For starters, buy equipment that will give you an overall workout, not just one body part; (2) buy equipment that provides many levels of resistance; (3) buy "spot" (for example, thighs, arms, etc.) equipment only after you've reduced overall and want to focus in on one body part. Before you plunk down your money, write up an exercise program you can stick to.

*I'll think long and hard before I make such a costly investment. Besides, I've been doing just fine with my gym shoes and sweat suit.*

# DAY 89

*What does the American Dream mean to you?*

The promise of riches has always been a part of the national consciousness. The American Dream attracts immigrants from across the globe in search of a better life. It's interesting, however, that the big Dream has always been defined in terms of money and the acquisition of things. In other words, it's about getting paid. Higher values like common decency, kindness, and loyalty are only valuable if they serve the bottom line. Don't get caught up in the madness. The constant, never-ending quest for material goods and money is a sickness that causes stress-related diseases.

*I know I need money, but I've got
it in perspective.
My big Dream is more about
achieving health and
loving myself than
acquiring things.*

# DAY 90

*Queen Latifah is the epitome of physical and intellectual strength and feminity.*

Latifah broke into show business as a rap artist. Now she's CEO of Flavor Unit Records and Management Company.[5] She's also an actor who, so far, has chosen her roles responsibly. Hollywood's depiction of Black women as mammies, prostitutes, and drug addicts has wreaked havoc on our image and collective self-worth. That Latifah's character Khadijah on "Living Single" is a strong Black *feminine* woman who loves and works with passion is a joy to behold. She never talks about going on a diet and, best of all, her relationships with the other women characters feel real; they depict the joys and trials of being true to the sisterhood. It helps us to see Black women characters that we can laugh with, learn from, and be inspired by. Go on, Queen!

*Queens like me and Latifah are rare, precious jewels.*

# DAY 91

*What the mind can conceive, the body will achieve.*

Some of us have been so heavy for so long that it feels as if we're permanently stuck. It becomes difficult to imagine ourselves as slimmer, fit, and healthy. Even those of us with only five or ten pounds to lose may be having a hard time. Now is when we must, as Jesus said, "become as little children." We must invoke our powers of imagination. If you can't imagine the shape your body is to take, how will you ever attain your goal? Without the ability to visualize your future body, your goal becomes a mere wish, a hope. Build those hopes and dreams into goals and commitments. Take a few moments each day to see your new, healthy body. Want to appear to lose a few pounds fast? Simply stand up straight. Imagine a rope attached to the top of your head, pulling you up straight and tall.

*I visualize myself as healthy, fit,
and energetic.*

# DAY 92

*"Girl, do you think I care what she said about me?"*

Why are Black women so hard on one another? Jealousy, back-stabbing, and gossip run rampant throughout the sisterhood. When a mother is struggling with her stubborn two-year-old in the grocery store, we shake our heads in judgment. If a woman has gone dateless for a time, we wonder about the quality of her femininity and her inability to keep a man. Before you condemn someone else, first ask yourself the question: Is my house made of glass? Who am I to judge anyone else? In fact, with the many problems facing our community, now is the time to support one another, especially in the arena of health and fitness. The chances of us improving our health greatly increases as we wrap around us a community of support. We might not get it from our bosses or our mates or the society at large, so we better start learning how to be more patient and tolerant of one another—regardless of hue, age, hair length or texture, religious affiliation, education, and economic or marital status. We need each other.

*I value my membership in the Black sisterhood, and I will respect and love other sisters as I am learning to respect and love myself.*

# DAY 93

*Keep hope alive!*

Jesse Jackson must have been talking about Black women trying to create a new lifestyle of health and fitness. How often do we lose faith in our ability to meet our goals? But health and a brand-spanking-new body are such worthy goals, we can never give up, no matter how many times we've failed in the past. We can't go back on our promises to ourselves. We're too precious. Would you give up on a child who makes mistakes in school from time to time? Of course not. Nor should you ever give up on yourself. The strength to meet your goals is within you. Close your eyes, take a deep breath, and find it.

*I believe in my inner strength.*
*I can do whatever*
*I set my mind, heart, and*
*spirit to do.*

# DAY 94

*"Girl, I got to lose weight for me."*

Losing weight for self is crucial, but let's face it, self is not always enough to keep us motivated. The truth is, to a certain extent, we're comfortable with ourselves. If it weren't for the constant pressure from men, media, and other women, we'd probably never feel enough incentive to lose weight or tone up. We've got more important things to deal with in life—or so we think. Let's put this business into perspective. Our primary concern is the health of our bodies, minds, and spirits. Looking good is a bonus. Look, this is war, and we have to have a "by any means necessary" attitude to winning.

*I've got to become healthy for myself,*
*but I realize that I may need help.*

# DAY 95

*"Girl, I can't stand her. She makes me sick."*

Jealousy is a sure sign that you're unhappy with the way your life is going. Some women just seem to have it all together: they're comfortable with their bodies, big or small; they've got nice clothes, houses, men. Well, if you want all that, what are you doing to get them? It's no great trick to hate a sister because she's beautiful. In fact, that's the lazy woman's cop out. Isn't it funny the extremes we'll go to to justify our hatred? "Men just like her because she's light-complected." "Naw, girl, they like her 'cause she's got that, you know, good hair." Oh, grow up! In the meantime, your spirit is being corroded, and don't think that doesn't weigh on your body. The answer to this problem is simple: if you loved yourself, you wouldn't have time to be jealous of other women. You'd be too busy having a life!

*The truth hurts sometimes.*

# DAY 96

*"Girl, I would exercise—if I could just find the time."*

We're all busy with work, children, home. Women have so many demands placed on them, so many needs to fulfill. Our exercise sessions are often a low priority on our daily lists of things to do. In fact, "No time" is our favorite excuse for not exercising, second to "I'm tired." The problem is not "no time," rather, it is poor time management. All of us experience time leaks in the day—time spent gossiping on the phone with a girlfriend, time spent watching TV. The truth is, you've probably got more time than you realize. All you really need is the desire and a good 30 minutes of heart pumping exercise per day. If, after you've honestly assessed how your time is spent in a day and you find that you really don't see where you can fit in a 30-minute time block, consider the following strategies: (1) wake up a half-hour earlier; (2) walk during lunchtime; (3) work out during TV time; or (4) break up the 30 minutes into two 15-minute or even three 10-minute blocks. If you're serious, you'll figure out a way.

*I'm serious. I'll make the time to exercise.*

# DAY 97

*Are your thoughts like a broken record?*

Remember record albums? There was nothing more irritating than an album getting stuck and repeating the same phrase over and over. Are you thinking the same negative thoughts day in and day out? If your thinking is in a rut, chances are so is your life. The problem with ruts is that even though they're a nuisance, they're sometimes more comfortable than doing what it takes to jump-start yourself out of one. For Black women on the growth path, ruts are unacceptable. The prerequisite for getting out of a rut is changing your thinking. Instead of waking up and thinking, "Another day, another dollar," thank the Creator for the privilege of life. Then ask for a good laugh. Make small changes—get your nails done or your hair cut in that new style you've been thinking about. Risk saying hello to that fine man. Play hooky from work and take the kids to the zoo. Enroll in a class. Read a different type of book. Try on a miniskirt. Go for it.

*I don't know how many lives I've got, but this is the one I'm living now. I'm going to do what it takes to have a fun, healthy good time.*

# DAY 98

*Diabetes is 33 percent more common among Blacks than whites. The highest rates are among Black women, especially those who are overweight.*[6]

Diabetes is no joke. Diabetics face a shortened lifespan, in addition to complications—blindness, amputations, heart disease, stroke, and kidney failure. This horrible disease can be prevented or kept at bay through exercise, proper nutrition, and weight reduction. You know if you're too heavy. It's one thing to love yourself no matter what your size, and it's another thing not to buy into the skinny hype. But if you're too heavy, *and you know if you are,* consider losing the weight. Even a small reduction, say 10 percent, can make a difference. Do it for yourself. Don't set yourself up to pay in the future.

*I don't want to be sick. I want to be well.*
*I just got my wake-up call.*

# DAY 99

*Make peace with your body.*

America is the most violent country in the industrial-ized world. Even though we abhor violence, we are also fascinated by it. Most important, we have not learned peacemaking skills. The violence that we commit against ourselves is the source of the problem. We haven't quite figured out how to love ourselves, so we engage in all kinds of violent behaviors against the self—smoking, drug and alcohol addiction, risky, promiscuous sex, and overeating. Our very thoughts need strict policing be-cause they are so violent, committing crimes against our self-worth. Loving the self is the beginning of making peace with our bodies. It's as simple, and as difficult, as that.

*As more Black women learn to love
themselves
and make peace with their bodies,
we will begin to
see peace reign in our communities
and in the world.*

# DAY 100

*Reward yourself for your successes—even the small ones.*

Pat yourself on the back! It's not easy to achieve difficult goals that you've created for yourself. But when you've accomplished even a small piece of a goal, bring out the confetti and pop the cork. It's time for a celebration. Get a pedicure or a massage. Go to a movie. It's very important to give yourself positive reinforcement when you do well. Lord knows, we beat ourselves up too much. Positive reinforcement will keep the momentum going and you moving steadily toward the next short-term goal. Not only will positive reinforcement keep your motivation high, rewarding yourself is a self-generated act. Motivation that comes from within is always the most powerful.

*Victory is at hand.
I now know I have
what it takes to achieve my goals.*

# DAY 101

*Can you taste your food?*

There's nothing worse than sitting down to a good meal, and not being able to taste your food. Your appetite is still alive and well, but the food doesn't satisfy. When this happens we usually eat more food. Stop and think for a minute. Do you actually feel hunger? Pause and listen to what your taste buds are trying to tell you. Maybe the flavor problem lies not in the food, but in your life. Maybe your days lack flavor, spice. Maybe you're bored. Maybe you're eating too fast or allowing too many distractions during mealtime. Whatever it is, don't make the problem worse by eating more. It would be better to go without for a day or so. That way you can learn to hear what your body's trying to tell you.

*As I risk spice back into my life,*
*mealtime will become a more*
*satisfying experience.*

# DAY 102

*Are you a talker or a doer?*

We Black women talk more stuff about getting our bodies—hell, our lives—together, but where is the action? You can do therapy, you can do positive affirmations, you can do research, you can do visualizations. You can do all those things, but if you don't apply what you've learned on a daily basis, all you're doing is paying lip service to self-improvement. You're not serious about getting it together. Talking a lot will not burn calories or tone muscles. Start hanging around with people who are committed to action and learn how they manifest their goals. You'll seldom hear them say, "I'm gonna start my diet on Monday." If they talk about self-improvement at all, they'll speak with passion about the benefits of healthy living, or they might share recipes with you or the latest research findings. It will be hard for the first couple of weeks, but stop talking. Start doing.

*Talk really is cheap. I'm
committed to action.*

# DAY 103

*"Girl, I can't get started in the morning unless I've had my coffee and doughnut."*

Right, and by the time mid-morning or early afternoon comes around, you're crashing. Sugar is insidious. It starts out as your friend—it tastes good, it gives you energy, it comforts you when you're sad or lonely—but inevitably, it lets you down. At the bottom of a sugar crash lies fatigue, irritability, and addiction. Sugar addiction is real. It creates a physical and psychological dependency. Sugar also increases the appetite. If you are a sugar addict, you need to greatly reduce your intake. Read labels. Sugar is damn near omnipresent. Food manufacturers want to keep you addicted to their product, so they pour the sugar in. Look for fruit-juice sweetened products. Better yet, satisfy energy needs and your raging sweet tooth with some fruit. A diet rich in fruit, vegetables, and legumes will take the edge off your addiction, because those foods are high octaine. Detox from sugar. Go cold turkey or gradually withdraw—whichever method your personality will allow.

*Sugar's no good for me. I'm giving it up.*

# DAY 104

*Flex those muscles.*

Women tend to be wary of weight training because they don't want to look like Mr. T. While some women who train to compete do indeed bulk up, it's probably not that serious for us. We just want to tone up here or there. If you've chosen weight loss as part of your self-improvement program, you'll be happy to know that working out with weights will, in the long run, boost your metabolism. Muscles burn more calories than flab does, even while the body is at rest. Weight training also builds bone density (thus helping to prevent osteoporosis). If you have a health club membership, that's fine, but you really don't need expensive equipment. To start out, buy some 3- or 5-pound dumbbells. Lifting light weights with high repetitions will tone and enhance the innate beauty of your body. There are a ton of books and videos that can get you safely started. Do your research.

*Muscles are beautiful and feminine.*

# DAY 105

*Women can learn a lot from men.*

Yes, it's true. Men have qualities that, if applied, can make us wildly successful in our health and fitness efforts. (1) Men are focused: once a man knows what he wants (for example, a female), he seldom loses sight of his goal. (2) Men are persistent: once a man knows what he wants, he never gives up. (3) Men are driven: the energy a man will apply to the achievement of a goal is a wonder to behold. (4) Men have a "by any means necessary" attitude: it's amazing to see the lengths to which a man will go to get what (or whom) he wants. Black women, let's learn from our dearly beloved brethren. After all, we know from experience how successfully they use these techniques.

*Men: you can't live with them and*
*you can't live without them.*

# DAY 106

*Don't quit!*

It doesn't really matter how quickly you achieve your health and fitness goals. What matters is whether or not you persevere until the end. The ability to push through fatigue, disillusionment, and fear is a skill that will help you in all areas of your life. Besides, there's no rush. In fact, it's best to take your time. Crash diets and frantic, sporadic workouts often result in added pounds, frustration, and binge eating. Slow, steady progress will ensure success.

*I am becoming stronger every day.*
*Perseverance makes me stronger.*

# DAY 107

*Prevention is just good common sense.*

Much of the attention we give to our bodies is done after the fact—after illness has struck, after weight has been gained, after muscle tone has been lost. Doctors prescribe therapies and medicines, and we grit our teeth to proceed. Wouldn't it make more sense to live the kind of life that would prevent these problems from occurring in the first place? For ourselves and for our children's sakes, let's start being proactive rather than reactive regarding our health. Let's eat nutritionally balanced, low-fat meals that are high in fiber. Exercise must not be avoided. The high-risk behaviors in which we occasionally indulge must be eliminated altogether. Visit your doctor periodically. Makes no sense crying tears and wailing "If only . . ." after the fact.

*An ounce of prevention really is*
*worth a pound of cure.*

# DAY 108

*Sixty-eight percent of Black babies are born to unwed mothers.*

While some may want to attach morality to this dilemma in our community, our main concern here is health—mental, physical, emotional, and spiritual—the health of black mothers and their babies. The stress of one parent (usually Mama) trying to raise a family single-handedly can wreak much havoc on the body, especially if there is little community or family support. Single parents who work often resort to fast food or frozen dinners. The loneliness of raising a family alone can be overwhelming at times; desperation often drives women to jump into bad relationships, which causes even more stress to the mind and body. In the midst of turmoil, it is of utmost importance that you find your center of peace. There you will find the answers to the challenges that are facing you. Even questions like, "How will I find time to exercise?" will be answered in that center of peace. If you can't find it on your own, don't be ashamed to get help.

*My center of peace allows me to stand strong in the midst of chaos.*

# DAY 109

*The journey of a slice of sweet potato pie begins with a single bite.*

Here's a biology lesson for folks who love to eat. Say you get a craving for a low-fat version of sweet potato pie. You take a bite. All you notice is the delicious taste, thanks to taste buds that detect sweetness on the tip of the tongue, but there are other equally important things going on. Digestion begins when you take that first succulent bite. Your teeth and saliva enzymes get busy; right away they start moistening and breaking down food. The tongue is actually doing double duty. It's tasting *and* pushing the food to the back of the throat, then down into the pharynx, then the esophagus. Wavelike peristalsis action surfs the food right into the stomach. It is then forced out farther down into the small intestine. The gall bladder and pancreas produce enzymes that break up the food into the nutrients that will be swept away into the bloodstream and carried to other organs and muscles for fuel. The indigestible material goes into the large intestine, and is eventually expelled. That was 28 feet of traveling your sweet potato pie just did.[7]

*I am thankful for such an efficient, ingenious design.*

# DAY 110

*And the word was made flesh.*
*—JOHN 1:14*

It's a powerful force that makes the word *flesh*. The power of our words on our bodies is just now beginning to be understood. We speak the condition, good or bad, of our bodies into existence. "You make me sick." "She's a pain in the neck." "He gets on my last nerves." "Eat your heart out." While there are nuggets of truth in each of these sayings—for example, stressful relationships can cause problems in the body—there is also a self-fulfilling prophecy at work here. Whenever you speak these negativisms, your body has no other choice but to listen and manifest them. The strong emotion with which we speak provides the power. It's time to take responsibility for your own words and your life. Learn how to turn negative sayings into positive ones. "Eat your heart out" becomes "I will eat for the health of my heart." "You make me sick" becomes "I refuse to give away my power. You may be hard to get along with, but that has no affect on my health or my life."

*My words are powerful. I will take*
*care of how I speak.*

# DAY 111

*Thou shalt not lie.*
—*GOD*

Tell the truth, now, how honest are you being with yourself? Sometimes we play mind games to make ourselves feel better, but the problems still exist. A common lie we tell ourselves is, "I don't know why I'm not losing weight. I'm dieting and I exercise." It's true, metabolism slows down as we get older, but it's still possible to lose weight. Exercise is the key. So if you walked around the block once this week or you crash dieted for two days, you're lying to yourself when you say "I'm dieting and I exercise." Weight loss requires sustained effort over a long period of time, not activity in fits and spurts. Here's another favorite lie: "I don't have any time to exercise." Do you watch TV? Do you spend hours on the phone gossiping? If so, you're lying to yourself. The health of your body requires that you start being ruthlessly honest with yourself, and this must be balanced with nonjudgment and love. Rather, use the truth to steer your life in a new healthy direction.

*To mine own self I will be true.*

# DAY 112

*"Girl, I wish I hadn't done that."*

Do you have any regrets? That's one of the worst feelings in the world, because you can't go back and change the past. Regrets cause depression and low self-esteem. All of us have had episodes in our past that we wish we could change, but we can't. Those of us struggling with health and fitness issues are often besieged by regrets. We eat to comfort ourselves, which, of course, leads to more heaviness of body and spirit. It's a vicious cycle. Forgiveness is the first step off the cycle. No matter what you've done, or what was done to you, forgive—forgive yourself, forgive others. Second, you're going to have to learn how to love yourself despite your flaws and past behaviors. Self-love is a toughie in Western society, but if you're serious about being healthy, you have no choice.

*I refuse to live in the past. Today is a new day, full of promise!*

# DAY 113

*Surrender your cravings to a higher power.*

There are bad cravings and good cravings. Bad cravings make you think your name has been written on an entire sweet potato pie. Bad cravings make you hear voices; food starts talking to you, seducing. Good cravings come from the body gently telling us what it needs. In pregnancy, good cravings become louder as the body of the fetus lends its voice to the body of the mother. We want to learn to listen to the good cravings. You can develop this skill by allowing your body to go into the hunger mode. That means denying your appetite the loud, bad cravings. As you deny them, they will get louder. But you're the master of your body. Tell them to shut up. Ignore them. Pray to be released from them. As hunger makes its presence known, the good cravings will start whispering, "Gimme some spinach." "I want some beans." "Don't drink that nasty soda—I want some fresh juice."

*I release my bad cravings. I hear the still, small voice of my body whispering its good cravings to me.*

# DAY 114

*Your attitude determines your altitude.*
—BISHOP T. D. JAKES

Let's not settle for mediocrity today. Set your sights high. Too many of us are merely functioning. We're settling for much less than we deserve. To get through the day, we often ignore a myriad of nuisances—aches and pains, even mild depression. Do you believe you deserve perfect health and happiness? That's the first step. You've got to know that this is your divine inheritance. Next, you've got to pay your dues. It takes time, energy, and effort to make an excellent body. Don't settle for less. Really go for what you want. It's your life and your responsibility. You are limited only by your dreams.

*If I shoot for the stars, maybe I'll hit the moon. Better yet, maybe I'll reach the stars!*

# DAY 115

*"Girl, what do I want breakfast for?"*

It's a wonder we ever make it through the morning. If the purpose of food is to fuel our bodies, then eating breakfast only makes sense. Black women are some of the busiest women on the planet. From the moment we wake up, we're up and running. Too often we're running on empty, though, which only makes us irritable and prone to overeating. Our resistance is lowered, and we run the risk of catching colds and other ailments. Lack of food also impairs our thinking. Several studies of schoolchildren have documented the link between breakfast and academic performance. We Black women also need to eat a healthy breakfast—that is, no greasy biscuits and fried bacon or coffee and doughnuts. Try instead oatmeal with fresh strawberries and brown sugar, low-fat whole wheat pancakes with fresh pineapple sauce, low-fat carrot muffins and skim milk, turkey bacon with scrambled egg whites and herbs, yogurt, or a power shake consisting of fresh fruit and protein mix. Breakfast in the morning will also help curb your raging appetite throughout the rest of the day.

*I'm going to be much more conscientious in planning, preparing, and eating breakfast.*

# DAY 116

*To hell with dieting and fretting
about my body today!*

Do you need a break today? That's valid—if you've been diligent about your self-improvement plan, that is. Take off today and just enjoy your life. Smell the roses. Listen to the birds sing. Don't think about losing weight or toning muscles or managing an illness. Just be happy! It's a delicate balance, diligence and obsession. Days off like today can halt the slide into obsession. If you give any attention to your body today, let it be pampered with a hot bath or massage. You deserve it!

*I'm taking a chill pill today!*

# DAY 117

*"Girl, she gets on my last nerves."*

It's a funny saying we Black folks have which, like most funny sayings, contains a kernel of insight. When we allow our nerves to become frazzled by some tedious relationship, we get irritable and anxious. Our stomachs become unsettled, our heads ache. Believe it or not, there's a better way to deal with stress. (1) Realize that you have allowed yourself to get upset. You need to confront and put an end to whatever's bothering you. (2) Exercise can dissipate some of that nervous tension. (3) Try natural relaxants like camomile tea and warm milk with a few drops of vanilla extract. (4) A hot bath with Luther or Sade serenading you can also do wonders.

*All my nerves are intact. I won't allow anyone to get to me.*

# DAY 118

*"Girl, getting some ain't what it used to be."*

In this age of sexually transmitted diseases (STDs), it is irresponsible, pathological, and suicidal to allow un-committed partners to put naked penises inside of your body. In a comedy skit on "In Living Color," a man at a clinic was grateful that he tested positive for syphilis. "I may go blind, I may go crazy, but at least I don't have AIDS." Actually, you don't want any STDs. Treatment for STDs like vaginal warts are painful, costly, and time-consuming. They can be prevented, so why would an intelligent Black woman put herself at risk? For love? Loneliness and desperation? Beware: While there are a good number of men who are using condoms responsi-bly, there's still that contingent of the brotherhood who continue to play Russian roulette with their lives. If a man gives you any excuses for not wearing a condom, run as fast as you can.

*My body is too precious for*
*uncommitted, unprotected sex.*

# DAY 119

*How serious are you about living a long healthy life?*

The life expectancy for Black men is 65.5 years; for Black women it's 73.9.[8] But as we increase our risky behaviors—drug and alcohol abuse, smoking cigarettes, gorging on high-fat foods, engaging in risky sex—you can believe the gap will begin to close. The lack of self-love lies at the root of all risky, self-destructive behaviors. Addicted people usually hang around other addicted people and this sick little community reinforces one another's negative behaviors. If you're really serious about getting healthy, you might have to do some uncomfortable things. (1) Get some new, healthy friends. Break up with that old gang of yours. (2) Get help. Talking it out with a professional is one of the single most powerful things you can do to help yourself. (3) Learn to love who you are, despite what you might have done in the past, despite the mistakes you'll make in the future. (4) Accept yourself for all your strengths and weaknesses. This is the first step on the road to recovery.

*My new life begins today. I'm going to clean myself up. My health is the primary goal.*

# DAY 120

*Can you afford to get sick?*

One of the fiercest public debates this decade has been on the issue of universal health care coverage. Conservatives say that the problem has been overstated and that the current system serves the country just fine. Liberals say that homeless, unemployed, and self-employed people are not being covered. Conservatives say that's their problem. Liberals say that compassion must dictate federal policy, not the bottom line. "The National Medical Association has found that 25 percent of Blacks have no medical insurance and 23 percent have no consistent source of health care."[9] Regardless of your political leanings, most of us would probably agree that the best insurance is learning about prevention and wellness. Go to the library. Read up on proper nutrition. And while doctors are important, don't depend on them to make decisions about your life. Be responsible for your own health.

*My insurance policy doesn't cost a cent. It's the Prevention Plan, and its all about living a healthy lifestyle.*

# DAY 121

*To create a diamond body requires time, pressure, and heat.*

The way Nature makes her diamonds provides a great lesson as we work to improve our bodies. Sometimes we get disheartened because the task we've created for ourselves seems so difficult. If you think your work is tough, imagine the birth and maturation of the diamond. One of the hardest minerals on the planet, diamonds are formed when carbon is subjected to great pressure and heat over long periods of time. To create a diamond body, exquisite and shining in health, we must also consider the forces of time, pressure, and heat. Since we are making lifestyle changes, we must have patience with ourselves. Re-creating our bodies will take some time. Our pressure is exercise. It will mold and heal our bodies inside and out. Exercise raises the heat in our bodies, which burns calories and flab. Diamond bodies are rare and valuable. Not everyone achieves their goal, because creating a diamond body is such a challenge. You're different, though. You can do it.

*I am a diamond in the rough.*

# DAY 122

*Are you a puppet, or are you a Black woman?*

Look, for the advertising industry, this weight issue is just a peg to hang profits on. Companies use high-priced beguilers to create the images and messages that keep you feeling insecure about everything from body odors to size to our nappy hair. And, of course, once they've created the problem they have the cure for everything that ails you. Once you begin to see that you've been used as a pawn in the money game you can't help but get angry. America has exploited Black people's lack of self-respect, self-acceptance, and self-love to make a profit. They don't care nothing about your childhood issues—except how they might relate to their bottom line. In particular, the fashion, food, and diet industries have greatly contributed to our unhealthy obsession with our bodies. You have been manipulated big time. So what do you plan to do about it?

*I'm going to start thinking for myself.*

# DAY 123

*If our society revered the larger, more voluptuous woman, what other reason would you use to put yourself down?*

Imagine big healthy women of all shapes and hues selling everything from haute couture to makeup to toothpaste to cars. Those kinds of images would create nothing short of a revolution in this country. Who knows? It could happen. Our spending power is as mighty as our heavenly hips. And what if it did happen? What then would you use to beat yourself up with? The size of your nose? Your ashy elbows? The point is, if you have low self-worth as a heavy woman in a skinny society, you'll have low self-worth as a heavy woman in a heavy society. Weight ain't nothing but a scapegoat for some deeper soul issues.

*I love myself, I accept myself, I respect myself.*

# DAY 124

*Are you reaping what you've sown?*

Payback is a mother, isn't it? The idea of consequences is an uncomfortable one, but eventually you've got to deal with it. When you were a child, you tried to get away with anything and everything. Some things escaped your mama's eagle eyes, but most things did not. When you grew up, for some reason, you forgot that for everything you do in life, there will be consequences to pay, either now or later. So if you eat a ton, then lie around the house, sooner or later your sins will catch up with you. Stop wringing your hands and moaning, "I don't know how this happened." Be honest with yourself, and never forget that you will eventually reap what you've sown.

*I will no longer play the victim. Today, I take responsibility for my actions, while accepting, loving, and respecting myself.*

# DAY 125

*Thoughts can be tangible things.*

Thoughts are things that manifest in the body. Slowly but surely, Western society is beginning to understand what so-called primitive peoples have known for millennia: thoughts are powerful, and they take flight on the wings of our emotions. Everyday, we must become more disciplined in our thinking and our feeling. Blacks are a creative, emotional, passionate people, and as we learn to discipline our thinking, our power will be a wonder for the world to behold. As we apply disciplined, enlightened thinking to our health and fitness efforts, we will become more focused, more centered, more secure in our belief that we can be successful. Guard your emotions. Don't let anything or anyone sap your strength. Guard your mind. Think high thoughts: self-respect, self-confidence, self-acceptance, self-love.

*My thoughts are literally*
*transforming my body and my life.*

# DAY 126

*Are you waiting for love?*

There's nothing like the love of a good man to make a woman feel that all's right with the world. If you have such a love, blessings be upon both of you. For those of us who have not yet been so blessed, are we going to wait around to live our lives? Too many single Black women, feeling desperate and lonely, resort to overeating and participating in unsatisfying sexual involvements. Overeating will only perpetuate a cycle of self-abuse and self-condemnation. Unfortunately, our society makes us feel less than a woman if we are manless, but it's time to change that. With the low numbers of eligible available men in our community, it stands to reason that many of us will experience solitude during some time in our lives. Instead of being miserable, let's choose to use these periods as a time for growth and introspection. Stop eating to dull feelings of loneliness. Allow yourself to feel all those uncomfortable emotions. Don't blow this opportunity for growth and real long-term happiness.

*I'm going to have a magnificent life, whether or not a man is in it right now.*

# DAY 127

*Can you take criticism?*

Sometimes the truth hurts, but hearing it may be necessary for growth. Some criticism is destructive, and your self-worth must be strong enough to know when someone's comments were meant to hurt. We're interested in the kind of criticism that builds up, rather than tears down. Criticism can be hard to take sometimes, because our egos get in the way. When someone offers you some *constructive* criticism out of genuine caring and love, feel your feelings, then try to put them to the side so that you can really hear what your friend is saying. It was probably as hard for her to share it with you as it was for you to listen. Thank her, and really take her words under consideration.

*No one's perfect.*
*I still have a lot to learn.*

# DAY 128

*When white folks catch a cold, Black folks catch pneumonia.*

Black folks make up 12 percent of the U.S. population, which makes us the largest "minority" group (although we're a global majority). Whites may outnumber us in this country, but we outdistance them in deaths caused by heart disease, cancer, strokes, injuries, homicides, diabetes, perinatal conditions, HIV infection, and, believe it or not, pneumonia/influenza![10] Why can't a people who were strong enough to survive the Middle Passage, slavery, and Jim Crow rise to this health challenge? Part of the answer may lie in this interesting piece of data: when heart disease rates are compared within income levels, rates for Blacks are *lower* than those for whites. Poverty is bad for your health, in other words, and one-third of our people live in poverty. The answer is clear: a prosperous people have a better chance of being a healthy people. First of all, we've got to obliterate our poverty mentality.

*I am a prosperous woman. I can afford to feed myself and my family fresh, nutritious foods.*

# DAY 129

*I love my arms.*

Arms are precious to Black women. They are the limbs we use to carry babies and stir up the pot, so to speak. We wave them about when we are angry and excited. They're always in action, always directing traffic. Keeping the arms in good shape is easy. Try this simple exercise, which you probably did in high school gym class: hold your arms out straight to either side. Do 20 circles to the front, 20 circles to the back. Feeling the burn? That's good ol' lactic acid. Carrying heavy grocery bags isn't enough to develop muscles. The secret to lean, strong, beautiful brown arms is working a variety of muscle groups in a variety of ways. Try using 3-pound dumbbells. Lift them in front of you, three sets of ten repetitions each. Take them out to the side, lift and lower. Do three sets of ten repetitions each. Bicep curls are also wonderful for giving you that strong, "don't mess with me" look.

*My arms are precious limbs, and I will keep them toned and strong.*

# DAY 130

*Nails should be beautiful and healthy.*

The days of cutting cuticles are gone. Manicurists have had to revise many of their practices because women were developing all kinds of infections. Cuticles actually serve a useful function. They protect the skin beneath and surrounding the nail from infection. Insist that your cuticles be softened, then pushed back—not cut. As for the many nail enhancing techniques, such as silk and fiberglass wraps, acrylic nails, and tips, long, strong nails are nice, but sometimes you should let your natural nails breathe. Go short occasionally. Every so often, do without the harsh chemicals.

*The point is healthy nails. As long as my nails are healthy, the natural beauty will shine through.*

# DAY 131

*"Gimme some fries with that shake."*

Black folks love potatoes—hash browns, potatoes au gratin, baked potatoes, mashed potatoes with gravy. Not only are potatoes versatile, they are a nutritionally rich food. They are high in potassium and vitamin C, so they are wonderful for people with high blood pressure. Eat potatoes boiled, grilled, or roasted. Baked potatoes are low-fat as long as you don't add the sour cream, butter, and cheese. Unfortunately, we Black folks love our potatoes fried, the greasier the better. Of course we can't continue to eat like that anymore, but that doesn't mean we have to give up our favorite food. We can fake out our taste buds with a baked version that tastes better than the greasy version. Simply cut potatoes lengthwise, season well with cajun spices or your preferred seasonings. Dab olive oil on them, and bake them in a hot oven until they're brown. Some recipes suggest brushing a thin coating of egg whites. Experiment. Use some of that famous creativity to make a better french fry.

*Thank God I don't have to give up my french fries!*

# DAY 132

*Once upon a time . . .*

. . . there was a woman named Ruth. She had two children and a husband, John. He wasn't the cutest or the most exciting man in the world, but he provided well for his family and he loved Ruth with a passion. About a year ago, Ruth started feeling restless. She began to feel that there was something more to life, but because she had it so good, she didn't want to complain. She managed to keep up a brave front, but almost without noticing over the course of a year, she gained 30 pounds. John could have cared less—he loved her, big hips and all—but she was appalled. Ruth began in earnest what became the greatest journey of her life: self-discovery. She learned she wanted to go back to school to study clothing design. And she wanted to start her own business. When she finally got up the nerve to tell John, he told her to go for it. As she worked for her degree, amazingly, without even trying, she lost ten pounds.

*Excessive weight gain is not only about food. It's about unrealized dreams, unresolved issues, stress.*

# DAY 133

*"Oh my God! Is that really me?"*

How comfortable are you in your own body? Here's a test: take off all your clothes, and stand in front of the mirror. Are you appalled? Can you stand to look? Try this: tell yourself how beautiful you are and say it aloud. How does this make you feel? Are you embarrassed? Do you feel sensuous about your body? Womanly? If your responses are negative, then you probably don't feel comfortable in your own body. Black women who are heavy or sick may engage in negative behaviors, like taking drugs or overeating, to disassociate from their bodies. Even sex can have an out-of-body quality to it. What you must do is learn how to be fully present in your body. This might require therapy, especially if past sexual, physical, or mental abuse caused the disassociation. Reconnection is absolutely essential to healing.

*My mind, body, emotions, and spirit form a healthy integrated whole.*

# DAY 134

*How much do you really want to change?*

We talk a lot about all the changes we want to take our bodies through, but do we really mean it? Have you ever made progress, only to backslide? There's something about change that's really scary. We might feel less than enthusiastic about our bodies, but there's comfort in the known—heaviness, aches, pains, and all. The change from a sick, unfit body to a healthy, fit one requires a major shift in how we view ourselves. This beginning mental and emotional work is absolutely critical to maintaining our goals once we've achieved them. We have to learn how to become comfortable in our new bodies. We will also have to adjust to the discomfort loved ones may feel as we make noticeable changes.

*I refuse to relapse. My mind holds
a clear picture of my new body.*

# DAY 135

*Time for a tune-up?*

When it comes to your health, don't procrastinate. Be diligent about getting checkups. Black women in particular can't afford not to visit the doctor regularly. If you haven't seen your doctor in more than a year, it's time to make that call. Black women are at risk for so many diseases, that it is absolutely critical we get annual checkups as a preventative measure. Pap smears and mammograms are a must. Regular visits to the doctor is a demonstration of self-love. Don't put it off. Call your doctor for a checkup today.

*I take care of myself because I love myself, and visiting the doctor regularly is one of the nicest things I can do for myself.*

# DAY 136

*Raise your expectations of yourself.*

Let's hold ourselves to the highest standard. Do not accept mediocrity in yourself or other Black people. We can do more than we think we can. If you've been doing well with your exercise plan, and you're beginning to feel just a little bored, now's the time to set a higher goal. Walk farther, run faster, swim more laps. If you can afford it, go on an adventure vacation. Climb a mountain, bike across a fruited plain. Participate in a walk-a-thon for a good cause. Challenge yourself more. Engage in a physical activity that intimidates you a bit. Surprise yourself. You'll be amazed at what you can do.

*I can do anything I set my mind to do. I will not quit.*

# DAY 137

*Your eating can affect your thinking.*

It's hard to think clearly when you've just eaten a five-course meal. You know the ritual during holiday gatherings—eat yourselves into a trance, and then fall asleep in front of the ball game. If you've got a big meeting or a test, keep your meal light. Fruits, vegetables, or yogurt can take the edge off hunger without weighing you down. If your energy level and mental capacities take a dive after lunch, it may be because you're either eating too much or the food you're eating is too heavy. The best rule of thumb is to keep it light.

*I eat lightly when I need to be at my peak mentally.*

*Are you satisfied with being just a piece of a woman?*

Western society can be characterized by its obsessive tendency to compartmentalize most things. For example, doctors specialize in treating certain aspects of us. So it should be no surprise to discover that many of us approach life the same way. Women feel they must deny aspects of themselves just to survive. We mask our sexual selves in a variety of ways, including work and religious service. Our little girl selves, the playful part of us, are hidden most of the time, if not completely denied. We are separated from nature and even other people. This lack of wholeness is completely contrary to the African way of existence. First peoples tend to view all of life as a whole within which the individual is a part. We can learn from "natural" women. Her work and worship provide all the exercise she needs. We need to integrate all parts of our lives. Work, worship, sensuality, play—they should all be one and the same.

*We Black women are multifaceted.*
*Our complexity is mind-boggling,*
*sometimes even to ourselves.*

# DAY 139

*Try a new workout.*

Cross-training is about adding variety to an exercise program. The purpose of cross-training is to exercise muscles that are being neglected by your normal workout. Cross-training also has the excellent side benefit of alleviating boredom. Let's face it, we get tired of doing the same thing day in and day out. When boredom strikes, we run the risk of quitting, and we just can't let that happen. A good cross-training exercise for walkers and joggers, for example, would be weight training. Aerobic exercisers might consider taking a swim once in a while. Yoga, tai chi, martial arts, and other mind-body disciplines are great, offbeat alternatives to most Western types of exercises.

*Cross-training makes sense. I'll vary my workout routine. After all, I can't afford to quit now because of boredom.*

# DAY 140

*Sweat is good.*

Funk used to be a good thing. A lot of us used to dance to it. Seriously, sweat is big business. The deodorant industry makes its fortune by convincing us that there's something unnatural, disgusting, even, about sweat. Sweat is natural. It's the body's wise way of ridding itself of toxins and balancing body temperature. Skin that sweats is skin that resists blackheads and whiteheads. Working up a good sweat is also great for releasing all that excess body fluid during moon time. Exercising, of course, is a great way to sweat (and remember that activity called sex?), but there are good, lazy ways to sweat, too. Sitting out in the sun (with sunblock), a soak in the hot tub, or a few minutes in a sauna will have you wringing wet. Black women have such beautiful skin naturally, and a good sweat makes it positively glow.

*I love that funky stuff.*

# DAY 141

*Sit up straight, girl.*
—*Your Mama*

Walk down any street in America and you'll see more Black women stooped over, as if the weight of the world is crushing them. Stand up straight! Hold that tummy in! The anatomical benefits of good posture are enormous, not the least of which is that it helps lengthen and strengthen the spine. There are other benefits, too. When we stand up straight, we're able to fill our lungs with more oxygen, which gives us more energy. Good posture is slenderizing. We just look better when we stand up straight. Equally important, the act of straightening the spine and lifting the head boosts our emotional and mental well-being. Even the slightest change in posture makes us feel better. We have and we project more self-confidence. We feel as if we can take on a world—and we can.

*My spine is straight, and my head is held high. I'm ready!*

# DAY 142

*Meat eaters,* beware.

Lately there have been reports in the media focusing on the questionable practices of restaurants and meat- and poultry-packing plants. The issue is cleanliness of processing and preparation. Because of inconsistent enforcement of FDA rules and regulations, you and your children are being exposed to toxic meat. Call it paranoia, but residents of Black communities should beware the meats they buy in their often inferior neighborhood stores and fast-food joints. There are a few things we can do to protect ourselves: (1) Do not suffer in silence. If you or your children get sick, complain to the restaurant or grocery store, as well as to the FDA. (2) Stop eating out so much. There's no way to know for sure how careful restaurants are in their cooking procedures. (3) Cook meat and poultry well. Undercooked meats containing E. coli bacteria and salmonella can result in death. (4) Purely for weight loss and health, limit your red meat consumption to no more than three ounces a day, three times a week. (5) Reconsider eating imported meat.

*I can do without the red meat.*
*I'll get my protein from poultry*
*and fish (well-cooked), beans, eggs,*
*and supplements if necessary.*

# DAY 143

*Time to jam!*

Have you wanted to include aerobics in your exercise program but couldn't get with the moves? It's no secret that our sense of rhythm is unique among the races. We are envied for our effortless ability to interpret a beat and a tune with the movement of our bodies. Mainstream aerobics videotapes and classes are highly choreographed and lack the spontaneity of a good house party. Well, there's good news. There are several new exercise videos on the market that have been made just for us. Featuring styles from hip-hop to African rhythms, they resonate with our culture and traditions while providing a serious workout. Or, use the creative ability you were blessed with. Turn on the music and jam! No more excuses!

*Funky aerobics? I like it, I like it!*

# DAY 144

*Is Black culture a fat culture?*

It's an unfortunate fact: Black folks are some of the heaviest people in the country. Why? Is there a fat gene in our culture? Yes! There are a few, in fact, because: (1) Our lives are too sedentary. We watch too much TV. (2) The transition from grease to healthy soul food cooking has been slow in coming. (3) The chronic male shortage in our community has led a lot of lonely Black women to overeat to deaden the pain. (4) We believe that any excuse is a good excuse for a feast. We love to party around food, food, food. (5) The identities and self-worth of many Black women are tied up in cooking and their love for feeding anyone who walks through the door. The last two points are not inherently bad. We just need to practice moderation. The first three points, however, need work. We Black women must begin to wield our power in our homes, faith communities, and neighborhoods. Obesity leads to too many diseases, like diabetes and high blood pressure, and unfortunately we lead the country in most of them. It's up to us. Let's fix this.

*There is much that is beautiful about my culture. I will use its strengths to build health back into my sphere of influence.*

# DAY 145

*Use a broom to whisk your waist away.*

Yes, the same broom you jumped over when you got married. The same one you use to sweep the kitchen floor. Simply put it across your shoulders behind your neck, then twist, 25 times on each side. Now slowly, lean over to the side as far as you can. Feel the stretch. Repeat on each side, 15 times. Now aren't you happy? You just saved hundreds of dollars on a fancy exercise toy.

*I love to stretch my waist and the rest of my body. The stretch feels good.*

# DAY 146

*Who gave* them *the monopoly on cute exercise clothes?*

Don't you just love those women who come prancing into aerobics class with thong leotards? And there you are, huffing and puffing in your oversized sweats. What they know and you don't is that cute exercise wear can provide a great psychological boost. You may not feel comfortable wearing skimpy leotards, but that doesn't mean you should go into class looking frumpy. It might sound silly, but a cute sweat suit might make the difference between sticking to your program or quitting. T-shirts with pretty colors or motivating slogans can help, too. Don't let the more advanced folks intimidate you. Huff and puff in your good-looking stuff.

*I always look good, even when I'm working out.*

# DAY 147

*Camera shy?*

Sometimes it's hard to tell whether you've made progress in your fitness program. The scale may be registering nicer numbers, your clothes may feel looser, and friends may have noticed and complemented you on the change, yet when you look in the mirror, you can't tell the difference. You're so used to seeing yourself in one way that the old memories of your body are blocking the real view. That can be a death blow to a fitness program. Soon you'll be thinking, "What's the use?" Keep track of your progress. Have a full body-length picture taken of yourself every two or three months. Progress is a great motivator, and with a picture as proof, you'll be less likely to backslide.

*I can't afford to slip up now. I'll do whatever it takes to keep me on track.*

# DAY 148

*Pinch yourself. Are you dreaming?*

If you want to know why you've allowed your body to manifest an unfit, unhealthy state, start looking at your dreams. They are a powerful tool for self-discovery. One of the purposes of dreams is to show us how we're *really* thinking and feeling about the world. Dreams remove the masks we wear in the waking state to reveal the true self. Only complete honesty about the inner life is allowed. Dreams may be difficult to interpret, but the more you work with them you'll be rewarded with a greater understanding of yourself and the ingenious ways your mind uses symbols. Dreams about food, for example, can tell you volumes about why you may be overeating, reasons that you may have hidden from yourself for a long time. Dreams about illness can be taken literally or they may provide a warning to change your lifestyle. Consider keeping a dream journal. Every morning jot down your dreams while they're still fresh in your mind.

*My dreams are an exciting path to health, fitness, and self-discovery.*

# DAY 149

### *Help!*

It's nice to have a buddy to help you through the big appetite/low motivation days. If your buddy is also struggling with health and fitness issues, however, your relationship will have some limitations. Misery may love company, but commiserating does little to boost self-worth and motivation. In addition to your buddy, consider finding a mentor to adopt you, someone who already has achieved her health and fitness goals and has been on a maintenance program for some time. She will have mastered many of the issues you are struggling with today. Seek out her advice, and be humble. Now is not the time for big egos.

*I will gladly sit at the feet of a master.*

# DAY 150

*Why are you a perfectionist?*

If you ask a perfectionist that question she'll say something like, "I just want to do a good job." If you do some probing, and peel away some of those rationale layers, you'll get to her core issues, which are usually based in fear. She's afraid of being found out. She doesn't want to be embarrassed if she fails, then everyone will know her shameful secret—that she's incompetent, or she's not pretty, or any number of things. Deep down, a perfectionist usually feels as if she's perpetrating. There's a lot of insecurity there. If this person sounds like you, understand two things: (1) you're destined for burnout and (2) you may be making life miserable for those around you.

*I'm going to take that chill pill today. I'm also going to find out why everything must be just so.*

# DAY 151

*Where's your sense of adventure?*

Are you the type of person who eats the same type of food all the time? If so, you are in an eating rut. If you have a tendency to overeat, the eating rut may be the cause of your behavior. You're bored, therefore you O.D. on the same old food in an attempt to experience a food high. The good news is that when you give your taste buds a variety of taste sensations, a little will go a long way. So try different ethnic foods (low-fat), eat at exotic restaurants, or try preparing your tried-and-true favorites in new and unusual ways. Come on, live a little!

*Eating exotic, low-fat, healthy foods is one of life's great adventures!*

# DAY 152

*The butterfly is a powerful, beautiful symbol of personal transformation.*

There's something wondrous about the metamorphosis of a caterpillar into a butterfly. Caterpillars, with their wormy, hairy bodies, are far from being the prettiest creatures on the planet. But then the magic happens, and an amazingly lovely thing is born. The beauty of butterflies, their wild, colorful patterns and light, quiet flight has inspired poets, mystics, and textile designers for centuries. As we struggle to metamorphose unhealthy, unfit bodies into healthy, fit ones, let's hold in front of us the image of the transformative power of the beautiful butterfly.

*The transformation my body is going through right now is beautiful and awe-inspiring.*

# DAY 153

*Clothes make the image of the woman.*

Let's do a wardrobe check. Whatever's in that bedroom closet will say a lot about your state of mind. Does your closet look like an ad for camp, with all the tent dresses you have in there? Are your clothes dark and foreboding? If you've been struggling with body issues for a long time, more than likely you've accumulated more than your share of dark, shapeless, lackluster clothes. What does your underwear drawer look like? Boring, plain white cotton bras and panties? As you move into a new phase of self-love and acceptance, you'll begin to grow restless with your boring closet. Manufacturers and designers have finally realized the huge, virtually untapped market comprised of women who do not fit the standard mold forced on us by the largely antiwoman image industry. So there is no excuse now to wear dark tents. Any woman can wear bright, outrageous colors with style and dignity. All the fashion taboos, like stripes, diagonals, and bold colors and prints, are being violated by beautiful women who have a love of self and a lust for life. Fabulous sexy lingerie and bathing suits aren't just for skinnies anymore. Whether you've decided to stay large, fit, and healthy, or whether you're on your way down the scale, look your best because if you look good, you really will feel good. Treat yourself to a fabulous, bold new outfit. It's a new day!

*I look marvelous!*

# DAY 154

*Too tired to sleep?*

Too much weight on the body can make us feel heavy and lethargic. Gallons of coffee and sugar-laden junk may temporarily boost energy levels, but inevitably you will crash. Barring any unforeseen medical problems, there are healthy, natural ways to fill your energy reserves. Raw fruit and vegetables will give you a great boost. Exercise, believe it or not, is better for you than a cup of coffee and a chocolate doughnut. Not only does exercise, especially the aerobic kind, release energy, it suppresses the appetite. How's your posture? If you're walking around with your shoulders slumped, not only are you blocking energy flow, you're sending messages to yourself, and to the world, about how you feel. Sometimes we're tired because not enough oxygen is getting to the brain. Deep belly breathing can give you the quick energy fix you need. Try it: inhale and inflate your stomach to a slow count of four. Exhale to eight, deflating your stomach. Repeat a couple of times. You should feel refreshed.

*I am a conduit for high-intensity spiritual energy.*

# DAY 155

*You're never too old to play games.*

Not the kind of hurtful games people play on each other, or the nonaerobic kind, like bid whist and gin rummy—we're talking active kid games. When was the last time you jumped rope with the girls on the block? Or played It? Or hopscotch? When was the last time you ran (or fast-walked) a race? Remember how much fun our games used to be? We could play from morning until night without the first sign of fatigue. Mama would have to call us in for dinner because we'd forget to eat. We never had to exercise because our play kept us fit. We never noticed time and we never felt tired. We were happy. We were energetic. We were hooked on the pure joy of playing. We can be that happy again. Roller skating, volleyball, basketball, jump rope—who was the killjoy who said we couldn't play anymore? Let's learn how to play again and just maybe we'll begin to adopt a more playful approach to all areas of our lives.

*Today I will play!*

# DAY 156

*Are you too good for your own good?*

Contrary to popular media depictions of us, Black women are some of the most conservative, moral people on the face of the earth. We are hardworking, often to the point of exhaustion. We give of ourselves and our money until there is nothing left to give. We would rather do without than steal. If we inadvertently hurt another person, physically or verbally, we suffer as much or more than the victim. We wrestle with our conscience on a daily basis. So when health and fitness experts tell us we've committed a crime by eating an occasional greasy french fry, we punish ourselves for the "sin" we've committed. We take Paul's admonishments about gluttony to heart, and our already low self-worth completely vanishes in the face of harsh self-judgment. We feel as if all the hosts of heaven are watching with knitted eyebrows as we eat that extra piece of chicken wing. Guess what: It's not that serious! Know in your heart that your value as a person does not depend on whether or not you met your health and fitness goals for the day.

*I am worthy! I am worthy! (Say this over and over while staring at your beautiful face in a mirror.)*

# DAY 157

*Access your body's original design of perfection.*

Imagine your body as it was originally designed. Reproductive, circulatory, digestive, and skeletal systems made up of organs, tissues, and cells—all designed perfectly. From the most minute details, such as the mood chemicals in our brains, to the melanin in our hair, skin, eyes, and genitals, we are a masterpiece, an amazing piece of work. *Every minute, old cells are dying and new cells are being reborn.* Unfortunately, the new cells are carrying over the new memories of fat or disease—not the original pattern of perfection. New cells are being created with the wrong program. Now, somewhere in our genetic code is the original Designer pattern of perfect health and size. It still exists within us! How do we access that original memory? Through exercise. Meditation and prayer. Nutritious eating. How about moral, ethical living? The Creator did not design us to fall apart by the time we hit thirty or forty years old, but that's what's happening to too many of us. Scientists who study longevity say that the human body has the potential to live at least a couple hundred good years. The Honorable Elijah Muhammad said 1,000 years, and the Bible says that Methuselah lived more than 900 years. Take a risk, and believe in the unbelievable.

*The original divine pattern of perfection lives within my body!*

# DAY 158

*Be responsible for yourself.*

We teach our children lessons in responsibility early on. We teach them to iron their own clothes, do their homework, cook their own food. We expect them to learn how to responsibly care for their own bodies by bathing and brushing their teeth. But are we teaching them how to care for their body by practicing healthy eating and exercise habits? How responsibly have you been caring for your own body, or are you still blaming people and past events for the condition it's in? You are responsible for your body's health and well-being. We can't demand of young people that which we are unwilling to do ourselves. That's hypocrisy.

*I'm no hypocrite. I take responsibility for the health of my body.*

# DAY 159

*Black folks lead all other groups in hypertension
(high blood pressure).*

And is it any wonder why? Think about what we've got
to deal with everyday. *Poverty:* According to the Census
Bureau, nearly half of all families headed by Black
women in 1990 were poor. *Racism:* Whites don't like
to admit it anymore, but racism, whether overt or subtle, continues to influence how much we make, where
we live, and the overall quality of life. *Sexism:* It ain't easy
being a Black woman in this U.S.A. Ask your girlfriend.
Ask the sisters who have allowed crack to completely
erode their moral foundation. Ask our ancestors. Ask
your Mama. The list goes on and on. Somehow, some-
way, we've got to learn to be peaceful despite the mess
all around us. We can do this. All it takes is determination and the absolute refusal to let anything or anyone
get in the way of your peace.

*I am like a mighty tree that stands
still and rooted in the midst of a
hurricane.*

# DAY 160

*"Girl, I feel like I'm being pulled every which way."*

Think of yourself as the sum of four parts: mind, body, emotions, and Spirit. If we were totally healthy, happy people, all of those parts would be working together in harmony. Unfortunately, most of our bodies are battlefields within which incredibly intense wars are fought. When it comes to food, each part has its own opinion and wages its own war about what, when, and how much to eat. The mind says no, but the body and emotions scream yes! The voice of Spirit can barely be heard amid all the noise. Call a truce. Let every part have its say. Ultimately, it really doesn't matter what they say. What matters is what you do. Your body and emotions may crave the whole cake, your mind may vote against even one slice, and the still, small voice of Spirit encourages moderation. If you can learn to be quiet, that voice will never lead you wrong.

*I live in harmony with all my selves, constantly striving for Oneness.*

# DAY 161

*"What is metabolism, and why don't I have one?"*

Metabolism is "how your body converts food into energy and then burns that energy as calories."[11] Yes, your body really does metabolize food, although maybe not as efficiently as it used to, unless you've remained active. Although you probably strongly dislike women who can eat anything and not gain weight, some of this you've brought on yourself. Flab slows down metabolism; muscles speed it up. We eat too much and we don't move around enough. Don't even think about dieting. It doesn't work. Only exercise will move your body into higher gear. *Age Erasers for Women* recommends the following ways to start your engine:

1. Step up the pace of your workouts.
2. Work out for longer periods of time.
3. Work your arms and legs more vigorously.
4. Exercise after you eat.

Also, stay away from stimulants, such as coffee, and consider having your thyroid checked.

*There's no way around it. I'm going to have to move this body.*

# DAY 162

*"Girl, I need that cup of coffee in the morning to get me going."*

Women with low energy can easily become addicted to foods and drinks containing caffeine. Coffee, chocolate, and some sodas are loaded with the stuff, along with sugar, and can cause health problems, like stomach ulcers, if constantly abused. Caffeine can increase your appetite, which is the last thing you need if you're trying to lose weight. It can also mess with your sleep cycle. If you're drinking more than a cup of coffee or soda a day along with caffeine-rich foods like chocolate, you're going to have to cut down for the sake of your health. But be forewarned: withdrawing can cause severe irritability and headaches. To ease the discomfort, wean yourself gradually. One cup of coffee a day's not going to kill you, but no more than that. Drink a half-cup in the morning, and a half-cup in the afternoon. Or mix your regular coffee half and half with decaffeinated. If you love drinking caffeinated sodas, try fruit juice–sweetened sodas instead.

*Cold turkey or gradual withdrawal, either way, I'm strong enough to kick the caffeine habit.*

# DAY 163

*Did you know that if you practice one conscious act of discipline a day for two months, you can create a new habit pattern?*

Who comes up with these rules? There is, however, some glimmer of truth here. Smokers: How long did it take to get addicted? Didn't you choke your first few tries? Drinkers: How long did it take to acquire a taste for alcohol? Chances are that first gulp of wine was awful. It took a few weeks of diligent use to acquire a taste for your bad habits, so it stands to reason you'll need at least twice that long to create new healthy ones, especially if you and your habit have been friends for a long time. Here are some practices worth making into healthy, lifelong habits: drink eight glasses of water everyday; exercise one half-hour everyday; meditate and pray everyday; and tell yourself "I love you" everyday.

*Good health is habit forming.*

# DAY 164

*Ever heard of a shero?*

We were raised on stories of men who fought wars and saved damsels in distress. They were heroes and provided great role models for growing boys. In the meantime, Black girls were raised on the stories of dependent, abused, beautiful Caucasian victims, like Snow White and Cinderella. Where were *our* role models, our sheroes, our stories about Nzinga, the African warrior queen, Harriet Tubman, the freedom fighter, and Ida B. Wells, the sheroic journalist? How different and empowered might we have been today had we been weaned on their amazing lives! Maybe we would be healthier, fitter women, too. Well, it's not too late for us or our daughters (and sons!). All of us—men and women, boys and girls—need to hear and hear again the stories of the great Black sheroes who, by empowering themselves, helped to evolve our people.

*I'm a shero to my self, family, and community.*

# DAY 165

*Do Black blondes have more fun?*

Black women have the right to do whatever they want to do. With that said, what about the latest blond hair rage? Is it right? Is it wrong? Black women who feel free to change their appearance in this way are often criticized for "selling out," for wanting to be white, for hating their own Black selves. But as Mama used to say, "Never judge a book by its cover." A Black woman who has dyed her hair blond may have a very strong, positive self-concept. Or she may be crying out for help. You'll never know unless you get to know her. Maybe she's just going through a phase, and tomorrow her hair will be blue. A lot of the criticism that is hurled against free-spirited Black women, daring Black women, is based on anger—these women simply will not be controlled. There may be some jealousy too. Secretly we envy the vivacious, uncontrollable wild women, especially if we are conservative, stable, and ultra-reliable. Let's hope that one day we'll reach a happy medium— wild, free women can learn from conservative women, and vice versa. In the meantime, though, judge not lest ye be judged.

*Nobody can tell me how to think,*
*dress, or act. If I continue to listen*
*to others' opinions, I'll never*
*discover who I am.*

# DAY 166

*Is your man or a loved one sabotaging you?*

Sometimes our worst enemies in the struggle for health and fitness are the people who love us the most. Whether because of fear, insecurity, or envy, it's often hard for them to watch as you work to become fit, healthy, and happy. The spotlight on you makes them look at their own shortcomings, and maybe they don't want to do that. So don't be surprised if folks try to make life miserable for you, even after you've talked to them about their lack of support. Don't get upset when they start waving the brownies under your nose, trying to tempt you. You may even have to part ways for a while. Your best move is to stay strong and focused.

*Success is the best revenge.*

# DAY 167

*Plateaus are a trip.*

You've been diligent. You've been working out and eating right. You've made a sincere effort to untangle yourself from bad addictions. Now you feel stuck. No matter what you do, the pounds just won't come off. Whatever you do, no matter how challenging the temptations, now is not the time to backslide. The body, in its wisdom, may need to stabilize itself at this particular plateau. Go with the flow. Allow your body to tell you what it needs. It really does know best. Don't allow impatience and desperation to force you into starving yourself or doing some other crazy thing. Be peaceful.

*I'll go with the flow because my body knows best.*

# DAY 168

*Might too much knowledge be a bad thing?*

There's such a heightened awareness of disease today—
particularly the diseases Black women suffer from the
most. A little information can be empowering, however,
too much attention to sickness and disease can cause fear
and obsession. The little hypocondriac within each of
us can grow to monstrous proportions if she is regularly
fed by the bad news media—new diseases and epi-
demics, conflicting information on causes and proper
treatment. It can get scary. We call for balance. For example, we need to know all we can about safe sex and
AIDS prevention, and caring people sympathize with
those who have unfortunately caught the disease. As
horrible as diseases like AIDS and breast cancer (pink
ribbons) are, we've got to keep them in perspective. Let
us study and put into practice all that we can do to prevent sickness and minimize the risk factors in our homes
and communities. Beyond that, our focus should be on
health and having fun in life.

*I will only think healthy
thoughts today.*

# DAY 169

*Does it make sense to have Black models advertise milk?*

Seventy percent of Black people are lactose intolerant, which means that the vast majority of us simply can't stomach milk. In fact, Whoopie Goldberg was supposed to do one of those milk mustache ads, but the National Fluid Milk Processor Promotion board turned her down cold when they discovered that she is lactose intolerant. Lactose intolerance occurs in people who lack lactase, an enzyme secreted by the intestines. Lactase helps to break down and digest lactose, the sugar in dairy foods. Some people are so sensitive to lactose that they may react to a slice of bread, which may contain small amounts of milk. If you love the taste of milk, buy lactose-reduced dairy products, or take lactase supplements. If you can take milk or leave it, get your calcium from other foods, like broccoli and kale, or take calcium supplements.[12]

*I'll get my calcium one way or the other.*

# DAY 170

*Black women are in serious need of inner healing.*

Think about all that we've been through since we landed on American soil. What a time we Black women have had in this country! From plantations to the projects, from slavery to welfare, we have had hell to pay in this country. No, not all of us are poor, but we can't deny that too many of us are suffering. Is it any wonder that so many of us are sick and unfit? Collectively and individually, we need to be healed. We've got scars on our souls, and they manifest in negative behaviors and debilitating body conditions. What we need is a love fest, a big party, a ministering service from Los Angeles to Harlem. We Black women need to purge the bad stuff and embrace love, prosperity, health, and sanity.

*I am healed. Black women are healed!*

*Leave me alone.*
—*You*

Oh, oh. It's that time of the month again. Premenstrual syndrome, or PMS, has been blamed for everything from spousal murder to cramps. "Up to 80 percent of all women report feeling out of sorts during the week before their period," says Susan Blumenthal, M.D., deputy assistant secretary for women's health at the U.S. Department of Health and Human Services. That's a lot of pissed off, whining women. Is it any wonder why men run? Why we run from each other? Hormones start tripping, and the next thing you know, you're pulling the wings off flies or ripping the head off some poor man. Consider trying the following PMS prevention tips to make life a lot more pleasant for you and those who are trying to love your irritable self: (1) avoid scheduling stressful events right before your period; (2) reduce alcohol intake, which can cause depression; (3) eat foods high in vitamin $B_6$, like potatoes, bananas, and broccoli; (4) get some sleep; and (5) if your symptoms are really awful, go see your doctor before you hurt somebody.[13]

*I turn the curse into a blessing by maintaining a healthy lifestyle and enforcing solitude when I need it.*

# DAY 172

*Intention activates the will.*

Intention is a most powerful action of the mind. Intention directs the mind and behavior toward a goal. When you decided to do something about the sorry condition your body was in, you directed your mind to resolving the problem. There was a shift from the routine "why me, I'm fat" type of thinking to "Damn it, I'm going to do something about this." Intention redirects thoughts and behavior and has them working in harmony for the good of the body. Intention activates the will. You become steadfast and empowered when your intention is clear and focused. You realize that you really can do anything.

*The power of intention moves from inaction to purposeful action.*

# DAY 173

*Oh, my aching feet.*
*—You*

A big part of the reason why so many people end up visiting the podiatrist has nothing to do with bad genes or accidents, and too much to do with tight shoes. Are we women still playing that silly game, the one that tries to squeeze a hefty peg in a skinny hole? Your feet are too important to be messing around like that. Don't mistreat them by wearing cheap, tight-fitting shoes. High heels are another problem. Whom are we trying to please? If a man can't love you in cute flats, then leave him alone. He doesn't deserve you.

*I look good and feel good in*
*comfortable shoes.*

# DAY 174

*Was that garlic or onions you had for lunch today?*

Some of our favorite foods seem to linger on and on. We're talking bad breath. Can't tell whether or not you have it? Well, if people are holding conversations with you longer than at arm's length, or if your man has been refusing to kiss you on the mouth, chances are you've got a problem. Fortunately, there's a nice little herb you can use to save your love life, and it's called parsley. That's right, that sprig of pretty green stuff that you usually push to the side at mealtime. After your meal, simply chew on the sprig. Parsley is so rich in nutrients, such as iron, vitamins A and C, calcium, and magnesium, that you should consider cooking with it regularly. A tablespoon or two in your vegetable soup or collards will also aid in the digestion.[14]

*Thanks to the humble parsley sprig, my breath is as fresh as a baby's.*

# DAY 175

*Get radical.*

Do radical stuff to prevent yourself from overeating. After your first helping, immediately put your napkin over your plate and say "Rest in peace" to signal to your brain that mealtime is over. Or quick, empty your plate in the garbage before you have a chance to think about it. Wrap the leftovers in foil right away and put them in the freezer. Black folks, no matter how wealthy, tend to have a poverty mentality that says "Eat everything, waste nothing." Take a bite, then run to the nearest homeless person and give it to him/her if you can't bear to throw it away or don't trust yourself to be disciplined. If you're at home or at work and can't give it away, put the food in the freezer, or force yourself to throw it in the garbage. Better there than on your hips!

*A crisis situation calls for radical action.*

# DAY 176

*"That girl knows she's got some big legs."*

Black women talk a lot about wanting big legs, but never do anything about it. There was even a song written in praise of the big-legged girl. Well, you too can have bigger, more shapely legs, if you so desire, and all it takes is a book. Not a small paperback Terry McMillan book, but a big, thick dictionary or encyclopedia volume. Now, put the book on the floor (not on the carpet) against a wall. Stand and tiptoe on top of the book. Lower your heels to the floor. Feel that stretch in your calves? Now raise your body, keeping your entire leg tight. Lower again. Do that 30 times every day. Your calf muscles will develop and grow, and your entire leg will benefit from the toning.

*Look out miniskirts, here I come!*

# DAY 177

*Self-love means self-forgiveness.*

Being honest with yourself is one thing, beating up on yourself is another. Sometimes we get the two confused. Being honest comes from self-love. There is no judgment or criticism—just clarity and desire to do better. If you've been beating up on yourself, you have probably not forgiven yourself for past mistakes. The lack of forgiveness can tip you over the edge into self-condemnation. Whatever you've done, forgive yourself, and just don't do it anymore. It helps if you smile in the process. Don't take yourself so seriously, and realize, we all make mistakes.

*I love and forgive myself.*

# DAY 178

*"I don't know if I'm ready to give it all up."*

Are you really ready to change your lifestyle from an unhealthy one to a healthy one? Do you really know what that will mean? It's not just about changing eating habits and working out. We're talking a complete life overhaul. Depending on what's going on in your life, you may need to do addition, subtraction, multiplication, or division. If you've got friends who are bad for you, subtract, add new ones. Multiply the amount of nutritious foods you eat, and you'll add to your lifespan. No time during the day? Divide your 30-minute workout into 10- or 15-minute blocks. You may have to subtract a boring, dead-end job and add a new one that satisfies your needs.

*This new math is a trip, but it works in making my lifestyle a healthy one.*

# DAY 179

*Use the pyramid for eating alchemy.*

Created by the ancient Egyptians, our African ancestors, the Great Pyramid at Giza has been transported through time and space and is now being used by the diet industry as a metaphor for healthy eating. The food pyramid is divided into five main food groups: You need six to eleven daily servings of the *carbohydrates group* (bread, cereal, rice, and pasta); two to four servings of *fruit;* three to five of *vegetables;* two to three of *dairy* (milk, yogurt, cheese); and two to three of *protein* (meat, poultry, fish, dry beans, eggs, nuts). Use fats, oils, and sweets sparingly. An eating program that spreads the groups across the course of a day will provide nearly all of the nutrients you need for health, longevity, and vitality.

*Diversity is the key to designing a healthy eating program.*

# DAY 180

*"I feel that as an African-American woman the only*
*thing I can do is continue to better myself,*
*continue to perform well.*
—JACKIE JOYNER KERSEE[15]

Jackie's the queen of Olympic track and field, with her
three golds, one silver, and one bronze. She is an inter-
national symbol of fitness. No one can deny her place
in history, yet even she feels she has more to accomplish,
more to strive for. We can always do better, push ourselves a bit farther. Obsession is not the goal. Excellence
is. We must hold ourselves and each other to a higher
standard.

*Jackie feels she's got more to*
*achieve, and so do I. Jackie and I*
*are high achieving Black women.*

# DAY 181

*They're trying to work me to death.*
—HARASSED WORKER

Ever heard of Blue Monday? Statistics show that heart attacks occur at 9:00 Monday morning more often than any other day and time of the week. Do we hate our jobs so much? Are our jobs literally making us sick? The stress of working with difficult people, doing work we hate, or being overworked is causing such an epidemic of backaches, headaches, and depression that it's a wonder the corporate structure continues to survive. Everyone's calling in sick! Absenteeism is high; productivity is low. It may be unrealistic to attempt to single-handedly change the corporate culture, unless, of course, you own the company. You can, however, change your response to the stressful climate. You can set parameters, for example, no overtime. You can go back to school to expand your marketability. Take your "coffee" breaks, but don't drink coffee. Stretch or take a walk instead. If it gets really bad, quit. You'll be amazed at how, when you take risks and obey your inner promptings, the Universe reaches out to catch you.

*My job is not worth getting sick over. My health and sanity come first. I will no longer put a job before my well-being.*

# DAY 182

*Pinch yourself. Are you dreaming, or are you planning?*

A dream can kick us out of complacency and into action. Dreams can be a motivating force awakening us from unconsciousness. Problems arise, however, when we stay stuck in the dream state and never get anything accomplished. "I wish I had a man." "I wish I was thin." "I wish my knees didn't hurt." "I wish I had some money." Rather than dream about what you want, you need to begin planning *how* you're going to make your dreams come true. Only you can move wishes from the dream state into manifestation. Don't get stuck in planning, either. You're going to have to *do* something.

*It's time to wake up. I commit myself to action. I want my dreams fulfilled.*

# DAY 183

*Do diet gurus ever gain weight?*

Every new fitness approach, diet, or exercise equipment has a skinny, muscular celebrity. The overkill is tiresome. Most of these gurus are blonds, and their body types rarely resemble our own. Yet, we buy their tapes, read their books, listen to their words of wisdom, and more often than not, walk away more frustrated than ever. Where are the beautiful, fit Black gurus? We need a bunch of them, and we need them in all shapes and sizes. Reality check! Close your eyes and turn inward. Become your own guru. Set your own standards. If you need outside inspiration, search out the ones who look like you.

*My own Spirit is my guru, and it moves me farther along the path to high, ecstatic states of health and fitness.*

# DAY 184

*"Girl, it's hard to get back in shape when you get older."*

But were you ever in good shape? Just because you were skinnier during your youth doesn't mean you were healthy and fit. Your metabolism was higher, so you were thin by default. Remember what you used to eat back in those days? Potato chips for breakfast, lunch, and dinner, maybe some fried chicken wings occasionally. Most kids hate beans and vegetables. Chances are, you did, too. Believe it or not, it is actually possible to be healthier and in better shape now than when you were younger. You now have the maturity to apply all that you've learned about health and fitness to your daily routine. You can actually become healthier as you age. All you have to do is apply yourself to the task.

*Everyday in every way I am getting healthier and healthier.*

# DAY 185

*Stressbuster: fish meditation*

We've got to get our tension levels and our blood pressure under control. Take a trip to your local pet store and buy a couple of blue neon fish. Put them in a peaceful spot in your home. Now, whenever you start feeling stressed out, look at the fish. That's all you have to do. The fish will do the rest.

*There's more to fish than frying.*

# DAY 186

*Declare your independence.*

Liberate yourself from greasy foods. Along with emancipation came the wonderful realization that we no longer had to eat like slaves. Greasy fried chicken, fish, and pork chops, salty junk food, sweets—no wonder we lead the nation in hypertension and heart attacks. Let's understand slavery in a different way. You're a slave to unhealthy living if you insist on overindulging in foods that are not good for you. Learn how to prepare fish, poultry, meat, and vegetables cleanly and healthily. For example, instead of throwing a slab of salt pork in that pot of collards, season with a little bit of smoked turkey leg or just herbs and spices. Let's not let our ancestors' horrific experiences be in vain. They were forced to eat what no one else wanted, and just barely enough to survive. We don't have to eat that way anymore. *And poverty is no excuse!* You can buy fresh fruits and vegetables with food stamps. As long as we are chained to unhealthy eating, we do the memory of our ancestors a disservice.

*I am free from the addiction of badly prepared low-nutritional foods. I only eat fresh, healthily prepared foods today.*

# DAY 187

*"Mine sure don't look like those."*

It's not always easy to be thankful for what you have, or don't have. America's image factory perpetuates the myth of large, perky, gravity-defying breasts as the standard, but as we all know, breasts come in many shapes and sizes. Gravity, the helpful force that keeps us planted on the earth, becomes malevolent when it comes to our breasts. Gravity, time, pregnancy, illness, age—we rebel against them all for the sake of perkiness. Women will willingly undergo the knife, risking their lives to lift and/or enlarge the breasts. We need to change this madness. There's nothing wrong with exercising that area to develop strength and tone. There *is* a problem with obsessing over a process that is as natural as breathing. Let's not be afraid of breasts that may hang low, singing sweet chariot. As Estella Conwill Majozo says, we "lactate from sacred spaces."[16] Our breasts must come to mean more to us than showpieces. They contain the milk of life. Check yourself periodically for lumps and bumps. If you're over forty, get your annual mammogram. Wear comfortable, supportive bras. But whatever you do, stop condemning yourself to a lifetime of despair just because your breasts have begun to s-s-*sag*.

*I love my breasts!*

# DAY 188

*What are you afraid of?*

Has this ever happened to you before? You've lost weight and, over time, you start getting compliments. Men suddenly begin to notice you. At first you're flattered, but something else kicks in, too. A little tempter voice says, "I'm doing pretty good. I can afford to binge just this once." The next thing you know, you're back to square one, and you have one more reason to dislike yourself: failure. The problem is not that you took a break, but that you continued to goof off. Could it be that fear disguised itself as the voice of temptation? Why are you afraid of reaching your goal weight? What will happen once you've achieved a fit, healthy body? To be sure, these are heavy questions. You may not be able to answer these questions on your own. You may need help. That's OK. There's no shame in talking it all out with a professional. *Whatever* it takes to facilitate healing.

*I question the voice of temptation:
Who are you really, and why are
you sabotaging my health and
fitness efforts?*

# DAY 189

*"Girl, I will hurt you if you mess with my slow jams."*

What kind of music are you listening to? We Black women love our slow jams, but do you ever *listen* to the lyrics? Some of them are downright irresponsible. They tell us we can't survive or breathe without a man. They tell us we're helpless; after all, we're only women. (Please!) The hypnotic beat only exacerbates the problem. We love our men, don't misunderstand, but we must love ourselves more. As this year is focused on building Self, we must look at everything that we see, hear, and feel that might be hindering our progress. Slow jams could be exacerbating your feelings of loneliness and depression. Listen to music that is inspirational. Exercise to it. Sing with it! Music can be a powerful tool for healing our bodies and souls.

*Upbeat, inspirational music lifts my spirits and motivates me to stick to my program.*

# DAY 190

*I love being a Black woman.*

We don't celebrate the fact that we're Black women enough. We need a national holiday—and Mother's Day doesn't count. We need our own special day that commemorates our magnificent selves. Black women are the backbone of many of our families. Often with little support, we do it all—we work, we cook, we clean, we nurture, we love. We're mothers, daughters, sisters, aunts, godmothers, grandmothers, friends, and lovers. We need some glory songs. We need some art that shows us sitting in a pile of roses. We need more visually beautiful movies like *Daughters of the Dust*. National Black Women's Day is our day for a collective pat on the back. We deserve it.

*Black womanhood is a national treasure. It's time we knew it.*

# DAY 191

*Is there truly such an animal as a fried chicken substitute?*

Fried chicken has come under serious attack by the nutritionists, and for good reason. Any food soaked in grease and fried is looking for an artery to clog. So it would make sense that we eliminate fried chicken from our diet. There's just one problem. Black folks love fried chicken. So what's a fried chicken lover to do? Oprah's cook Rosie Daley and many others have created reasonably decent fake fried chicken recipes that are really baked. The success of fake "fried" chicken depends on an abundance of seasoning (minus the salt), ice-cold water, and cooking spray. Rosie also uses nonfat yogurt.[17] Give it a try. Do your research. Better yet, experiment. Who knows? You might like it better than the greasy version.

*I'm a cooking genius. I can even make fake fried chicken taste good.*

# DAY 192

*Exercise your inner sight for early warning signals.*

Inner sight is a tool of the imagination and spirit within us. Inner sight involves visualizing the cells, tissues, and organs in as much detail as possible. Amazingly, symbols, colors, or even feelings may come to mind as you scan certain areas. To help your imaginative powers, take a look in a children's anatomy book. Look at the shape, color, and details of the various organs. Look at your own body. Touch and memorize the shape, color, and texture of your fingers, elbows, knees—all your extremities. Now close your eyes. Move your inner sight throughout your body, from your hair to your toes. Go from body part to body part. See your arms, breasts, heart, pancreas, vagina. Try to feel them. Rest upon an area that might be cause for concern, and wait for your body to tell you, in its own unique way, what's going on there. You might see a color, or a symbol, or a scene of some sort. Don't look to others to interpret what you've seen. Ask your body. And by all means, if you perceive a warning, consult your doctor immediately.

*Learning about my body through inner sight is an excellent way to assume responsibility for my health.*

# DAY 193

*FAT FACTS: All oils are 100% fat.*
*One tablespoon of oil equals 120 calories.*
*Some fats are better for you than others.*

Before you do anything else, you've got to do one thing that could save your life. THROW THE LARD IN THE GARBAGE! Lobby for its removal from your local grocery store. Animal-derived oils, that is, saturated fat, are increasingly being blamed for clogged arteries, heart disease, and a shortened lifespan. Cook with as little oil as possible, but when you must use oil, use vegetable-based mostly monounsaturated oils, like canola, sunflower, safflower, soybean, and olive. They contain vitamin E and less of the bad stuff.

*I'm going to start cooking smarter*
*with healthy oils.*

# DAY 194

*Power is activated when you accept that you have it.*

The most important factor in successfully pursuing health and fitness is an unswerving belief in yourself. You have to know that you can do this thing. You have to believe it with all your heart, you have to know it with your mind, you have to feel it in your body. Let your spirit empower your belief and give direction to your activities. You really can do this. You are more powerful than you could ever imagine.

*I accept and use my spiritual power to heal myself and feel whole.*

# DAY 195

*What is love?*

Everyone agrees we must love ourselves, but no one can agree on what love is. Here we offer yet a new definition: Love is a state of being. Certain emotions and activities proceed from the love state. We often confuse emotions, like passion, and activities, like gift giving, with love. Emotions and activities may or may not determine a love state. So how do you know if you love yourself? If you love yourself you may feel warmth in your heart. A smile may touch the lips when you look at yourself in the mirror. Or, you may do positive, life-affirming things, like eating right and exercise. Most important, however, self-love is a state of being that creates harmony among mind, emotions, body, and spirit. Loving oneself is so very hard to do, but if we are to build motivation from within, it is absolutely imperative to allow Love to manifest as a constant, dependable state of being.

*My love for myself is more than an emotion or a pedicure—my self-love manifests as harmony and peace.*

# DAY 196

*I've got the arms, honey, and the abs. It's my legs I've gotta work on.*
*—ANGELA BASSETT*[18]

Granted, playing Tina "Legs" Turner must be an incredibly intimidating task, but Angela! Have you looked in the mirror lately? Your legs are fabulous! Just as they are! Angela Bassett trained hard for her role in *I, Tina,* and has the body to show for it. Not an ounce of flab anywhere. Yet, there's still the feeling that something's wrong. At what point in our fitness plan do we say, "It is finished. I am pleased with my body"? Don't let a quest for perfection prevent you from patting yourself on the back if you've worked hard.

*I will rethink my quest for perfection and accept every stage of my development as perfect for the time.*

# DAY 197

*Don't quit!*

Sometimes we feel like quitting our eating or exercise program because they've become boring. One egg white for breakfast, tuna fish and crackers everyday for lunch just ain't getting it. The best antidote for boredom is fun. Put some fun in your food and workout sessions. Make a beautiful salad with a variety of lettuce leaves and edible flowers. Walk backward instead of forward. Play like a kid again. Look for fresh approaches to your food program or workout routine. You'll become stronger and more disciplined, and you might even have some fun.

*Fun is the new ingredient in my
health and fitness program.*

# DAY 198

*Taking a trip?*

Why is it we forget all about our eating program when we're on vacation? It's as if fat grams and calories don't count in foreign ports of call. Cruise ships in particular are notorious for their orgies of feasting. No way could we be expected to exercise restraint on a cruise ship. We're on vacation, after all! Ah, but the debt will be paid, dear sister. All that hard work that got you into bathing suit readiness will be all for naught. You'll come home bigger than when you left. Here's a strategy: don't gorge yourself, sample instead. Try a variety of cuisines, but in small portions. Walk, swim, or take aerobics classes daily. If you're serious about your program, not even a vacation will take your eyes off the prize.

*Calories and fat grams do count, whether at home or in a faraway land. Restraint and enjoyment are balanced and I am able to stick to my program while enjoying life.*

# DAY 199

*Grow your own herbs and vegetables.*

There was a time when our ancestors lived totally off the land. For those of us whose needs are met by the corner grocery store, it is difficult to imagine actually growing food and foraging for medicinal herbs. Granted, times have changed, but the human need to connect to the soil will always be a dynamic within us. Equally important is the satisfaction that comes from consuming what you have produced. Whether you live in a tiny urban studio or are a homeowner, you can grow herbs and even some vegetables, and you can grow them organically, without pesticides. If you're an apartment dweller, try growing herbs like basil, mint, thyme, and parsley in pots. Aloe plants thrive indoors, and the gel is wonderful for soothing minor burns. For those who have access to even a tiny plot of land outdoors, try growing tomatoes, cucumbers, broccoli, bell and jalepeño peppers, eggplant, collards, cabbage, and celery.

*Growing my own food empowers my pocketbook and enables me to take direct responsibility for my health.*

# DAY 200

*"Girl, ain't nobody sticking no needles in this here body."*

Alternative therapies are becoming more acceptable in our culture. Contrary to the West's preoccupation with invasive and drug-based techniques, alternative therapies naturally activate the body's own healing mechanisms, and they work on the whole person. For example, different bodyworking technologies, such as rolfing or network chiropractic, not only seek to realign the spine and knead out the rough spots in the muscles and joints, but in the process, past memories are often released from areas within which they may have been lodged for years. Acupuncture (and acupressure) is an ancient Chinese therapy that unblocks the flow of energy in ailing body parts with needles or pointed, targeted pressure. Aromatherapy is gaining credibility as a healing technology through scent. Music, dance, and art therapies use the untapped creative aspects of us to understand and heal underlying problematic behaviors and emotions. Consider using alternative therapies along with traditional Western treatment.

*I am open to new ideas about health, healing, and fitness.*

# DAY 201

*Are you waiting for the rapture?*

When life gets too overwhelming, the natural human response is to look for a way out. If we can't see our way clear, we get to praying. "Oh, Lord, send the Messiah today!" Be honest. Do you want the End of Time to occur because society is sick and needs a cleansing, or are you looking for a way out of your misery? A lifetime of bad habits and bad decisions have possibly brought you to this point, and it's time to pay up. Take heart, you're not alone, nor are you weak and ill-equipped. What kind of Black race of people will meet the new millennium? Will we be strong, healthy, and ready to assume our rightful place in the global scheme of things, or will we be fat, sick, out of shape, and looking for someone to save us? We must answer these questions with self and communal love and hope for the future. We can meet 2001 a healthy, strong people. It starts with you.

*In the twinkling of an eye, I can proceed from this new attitude: ain't nobody going to clean up my mess but me. I can do this.*

# DAY 202

*No more blaming the white man.*

We should never excuse, nor forget, slavery, Jim Crow, and institutional racism, but will blaming the white man heal you or help you lose weight? White people are the healthiest people in the country, and Black people are some of the sickest. We all have access to the same information. Why are we still sick? What's preventing the connection to occur between knowledge and smart behavior? For example, by now (unless you've been living on Venus) everyone knows that a cigarette is death on a stick. Yet Black people die from lung cancer more than any other racial group. We spend millions on cigarettes each year. *Why?* is the question to which we must give serious consideration. We are a smart race of people. Let's start applying ourselves to raising the standard of health in our communities. C'mon now, the white man's not physically forcing you to drink, smoke, overeat, and have promiscuous unprotected sex, although they may make it appear very cool. Irresponsible advertising may have stimulated a national climate of conspicuous consumption to which we appear most susceptible, but it's good to know the final decision and power rests with us.

*I alone am responsible for the condition of my body. I am empowered.*

# DAY 203

*"Oh, my aching back!"*

Chronic back pain devastates millions of people in America each year. The usual response is to take a couple of aspirin and lie down until the pain subsides. Others suffer so badly, surgery is required. The good news is that there are drug-free ways to take control of the health of your back. Make sure your diet is rich in calcium to strengthen and build density into the 26 bones that make up the spine. If PMS and menstruation is the source of your back pain, try a colonic or therapeutic massage, both of which can help alleviate some of the pressure off the spine. As pregnant women can testify to, a big tummy can make life hell for the lower back. Sit-ups help to reestablish strength and alignment. There are several asanas (poses) in yoga specifically designed to strengthen the back. Consider giving up those high heels. They're throwing your posture and alignment completely off center. You'll still look fabulous in flats. And finally, assess the condition of your bed and favorite chairs. They may need more firmness and support.

*The health of my back is worth the extra effort. My back is straight, healthy, and pain-free.*

# DAY 204

*Cranberries are womanfruit.*

As usual, our Mamas and Grandmas were right. *First* magazine cites research from Harvard Medical School that says that drinking cranberry juice can help prevent bladder infections.[19] Postmenopausal women who drank one 10-ounce glass of cranberry juice cocktail daily reduced urine bacteria by more than 50 percent. They also developed fewer infections. Sure, you know this stuff, but have you made cranberry juice, even cranberry muffins, a part of your healthy-eating, disease prevention plan?

*I will connect knowledge to positive proactive behavior. I will make it a point to drink one 10-ounce glass of cranberry juice a day.*

# DAY 205

*Let's have a new appreciation for okra.*

Okra is a soul food blessing. This humble vegetable is a nutritional powerhouse, packed with enough fiber to help prevent irritable bowel syndrome, chronic constipation, and colon cancer. It may lower cholesterol and stabilize blood sugar levels in diabetics.[20] Okra comes fresh, frozen, and canned—fresh and frozen are best. Okra is great in, of course, gumbo, but it works equally well in stews, casseroles, and whatever else your creativity can devise. Just don't overcook to limpness.

*Okra is now and henceforth a respected member of my food program.*

# DAY 206

*"Girl, I hate putting my feet up in those stirrups."*

Pap smears are like taxes: you can't live without them. As a prevention and early warning tool for cervical cancer, it is still the best medical test money can buy. Just a few minutes in the stirrups once a year (or as otherwise recommended by your gynecologist) is well worth the minor discomfort. Just lie down and relax. As you're lying flat on your back, imagine yourself sipping fruit juice on a beach in the Caribbean. Do deep breathing. If you haven't made that appointment yet, do it today.

*Pap smears are a necessary nuisance. I'll endure the procedure for peace of mind.*

# DAY 207

*Vesta's secret to weight loss: Transform a negative situation or event into positive motivation.*

When singer Vesta lost her recording contract, she knew that her size 24 frame was to blame. The harsh reality of the music industry upholds an unrealistic body standard for its successful female singers. Well, instead of getting depressed, Vesta got busy. *Jet* magazine reports that she lost almost 100 pounds in less than a year—with the help of a personal trainer and a total revamping of her food program. "In the beginning, I had a lot of carbohydrates and almost no fat. I ate lots of pasta, potatoes, and rice," she says.[21] In addition, Vesta eats salads and fruit and drinks water and iced tea. Red meat was completely eliminated from her diet, but she got to have her occasional fried chicken fix, just not as often as she used to. As with most of us, the whole weight issue is a sensitive one, and for Vesta, the pain was compounded because of her life in the spotlight. She turned it around, though, and for that we say, "Go on, girl!"

*Vesta's a lot like me: we're both strong, beautiful Black women who are committed to maintaining a healthy lifestyle, and achieving our goals.*

# DAY 208

*How are those orgasms?*

If you'd like better ones, you can strengthen your muscles with the famous Kegel exercise. Breathe in slowly and clench the vaginal muscles, as if you were holding back urine. Hold for about five seconds. Breath out and release. Do this a few times every day. The great thing about this exercise is that you can do it anywhere—in the privacy of your home or in a room full of people.

*Oh, yeah, clench, two, three, four.*
*I love my Kegel exercises.*

*Olive Oyl could learn a thing or two from Popeye.*

Our ritual loss of blood each month creates a craving within our bodies for iron. Women who exercise are also more susceptible to a tremendous loss of iron.[22] Iron-deficient women tire out easily. Women usually need about 18 milligrams of iron per day. Our need is high, yet even the most iron-rich foods, like spinach (one cup) or red meat (three ounces) only provide 2 milligrams of iron. Talk to your doctor about the possibility of taking supplements. (You don't want to overmedicate. Too much iron can be toxic to the body.) Eat iron-rich foods, like chicken liver, spinach, and beans. Also important to know is that certain foods, when eaten with iron foods, can either enhance or block absorption of iron into the bloodstream. You're going to have to do your homework, but here's a start: foods rich in vitamin C, like oranges and broccoli, will enhance iron absorption.

*Iron-rich foods make me stronger and give me energy.*

# DAY 210

*Black beauty is skin deep.*

Black women are richly blessed with durable melanin-rich skin. Through the harshness of life, a polluted environment, and bad diets, our skins miraculously withstand the tests of time. Look at the skins of many of our elder beauties. Elastic, firm, soft, black coffee to cream skins. We've got it going on, and, you better believe, we are envied. Just look at the billion-dollar industry that has arisen out of the desire to attack early and advanced signs of aging. Black women often don't manifest wrinkles until we're well into our 40s, even 50s and 60s. That's a blessing that should not be taken for granted. Now, harsh living will eventually take its toll, no matter a woman's melanin abundance. Alcohol and drug abuse, cigarette smoking, and severe stress can mar Black skin's natural beauty. Eat healthy foods, drink lots of water, get plenty of sleep, use gentle cleansers, and best of all, sweat. Our skin loves the sweat the exercise produces.

*My health and beauty are
skin deep.*

# DAY 211

*Don't you know that you are a god?*
—*JESUS*

Before Western civilization was the dominant global culture, Black women were revered as goddesses. Our images have been found on archaeological digs all over the world. Images of full breasts and wide, rolling hips have been immortalized in stone and wood. That is your heritage. The Afrocentric movement has blessed us with a powerful image that is very important in the discussion of body image: the image of the African queen. Most of us were raised on the histories and legends of European kings and queens. We, too, come from an ancient continent of kings and queens, many of whom were known for great physical beauty, strength, and mental prowess. Nefertari, Esat, Cleopatra, Nefertiti, Nzinga, and Sheba—they were the Black queens after whom African women patterned themselves. *These* magnificent women were the standard. So how do we understand the African queen in light of our health and fitness efforts today? We internalize the queen as the ruler of the self. The power and beauty of the queen is in our genetic code. It's in us, just waiting to rule in our lives.

*I am the new standard*
*of beauty. (Affirm this to yourself*
*throughout the day.)*

# DAY 212

*Don't spend good money on an expensive weight set!*

Milk cartons will serve just as well in the war against flab. Buy two plastic quart containers (with handles) of skim milk. Rinse out the empty cartons and fill both with water about a quarter of the way up. Grasp the handles, and hold your arms straight out to the side; raise and lower ten times. Now hold your arms straight out in front of you; raise and lower ten times. Once again, extend your arms straight out to the side; holding your arms straight, close them in front of your chest, squeezing chest muscles tightly. As you can see, anything you do with weights you can do with milk cartons, all for about $3. As your strength increases, simply fill the containers with more water. When you get really good and strong, you might want to invest the big bucks into a couple of gallon-size milk containers.

*Undermining the system is fun. I don't have to spend a lot of money to become fit.*

# DAY 213

*"Girl, I was so bad last night."*

Sometimes doing bad stuff like taking drugs or having unprotected sex, just makes us feels good. The hitch is that they're temporary fixes. Worse, they can lead to addiction, disease, danger, and death. The need for stimulation is a natural one, so go for the natural high. Listening to inspirational music, attending a faith service, having wild and crazy protected sex with a committed, monogamous partner, engaging in rigorous exercise, or reading a steamy romance novel or essay of cutting edge ideas are all safe, healthy, exciting ways to get an adrenaline rush.

*When the urge to do something dumb hits you, take a deep breath, close your eyes, and picture this: You're standing at the edge of a cliff that overlooks the most beautiful meadow you've ever seen. Jump up, stretch your arms and fly over the meadow. Feel the rush of air across your body. Hear the wind. Smell the wild roses. Now lower yourself to the bank of a clear, warm Jacuzzi-style brook. Take off all your clothes and step in. The rest of this fantasy is up to you.*

# DAY 214

*Take your vitamin.*
—Your Mama

Easy for her to say. When you were growing up, taking your vitamins was a simple affair. All you had to do was pop one candy multivitamin in the mouth at breakfast. It was like health insurance—just in case you didn't eat broccoli that day. Today, you need a Ph.D. to make your way through the maze of amino acids, antioxidants, and bioflavonoids. Let's keep it simple. Take one multiple a day (on a full stomach). If you're feeling tired, you might need an additional iron supplement to compensate for monthly blood loss; if you don't drink milk, consider taking calcium. Of course, your best bet is to eat a wide variety of nutritious foods—beans, fruit, veggies, and grains—but more than likely, we're not going to get everything we need from the foods we eat. So, like your mama told you, take your vitamin.

*I will take my vitamins every day.*

# DAY 215

*Is there such a thing as the "ideal" weight?*

As long as you're allowing outside forces to determine the right size for your body, you'll never have any peace. Whether your ideal comes from the old (even the revised version) and highly unrealistic Metropolitan Life Insurance Table, the latest fashion model, or Loquisha down the street, the point is, you're not being self-directed. Aren't you tired of the endless chase for a size that may or may not be right for your body type? Take your eyes off the world and begin to appreciate the body you were blessed with. Let your body guide you. Develop a communicative relationship with your body. Learn to listen to it. Hear the rage when you deny it food, the discomfort and depression when you overeat. Pay attention and heed. What does it all mean?

*When my body talks, I will listen.*

# DAY 216

*Don't you want to be free forever?*

Imagine a morning, unlike any other morning. You awaken, stretch, and sunlight beams through the bedroom curtains. You get up, take a shower, and—hold it! Something's missing. There's something you forgot to do. The scale! You forgot to weigh yourself! You look at yourself in the mirror, turn to the side, pat your stomach and hips, and—wait! You forgot to criticize yourself for overeating last night! Could it be that you're finally free? What a great feeling! If you haven't reached the Promised Land yet, don't despair. You will. Just hold that feeling in your thoughts and freedom from food abuse will surely come to pass.

*Free at last, free at last!*

# DAY 217

*Go for it.*

Give yourself permission to be the best you can imagine yourself to be. Set your sights high, and keep your eyes starward. Let there be no mediocrity in your life. Mediocrity is boring. Don't straddle the fence. Don't accept ailments in your body or situations in your life because they're bearable. If they are not bringing you health, peace, and joy, GET RID OF THEM! Use your Black woman courage, the same your ancestors used to get through slavery. They often didn't have a choice, and when the opportunity came, they fought for their freedom. You can do no less.

*I choose life, health, and happiness.*
*I'm going for it!*

# DAY 218

*Allow yourself grieving time.*

The loss of a loved one, a terrible accident, the loss of a job, divorce, abandonment—these incidents too often fill the lives of Black women, causing us untold stress, illness, and depression. Food, either eaten in excess or not at all, often becomes the symbol of our suffering. Fluctuations in appetite are normal during catastrophic times. But don't let it go on too long. Get help if the problem seems to be lingering.

*I will cry and talk it out for as long as it takes in order to reenter the land of the living.*

# DAY 219

*Do you have a secret place?*

We all need a special place in the world that we can call our own. It's a place where we can go to be left alone in peace. Solitude and quiet are welcome friends in the secret place. Find a prayer room in your home, your garden, a spot by the beach, or a cave at the foot of a mountain. Use this secret place to dream your dreams, set your goals, make your plans. Meditate and pray here. Heal here. Be very selfish about this secret space. Sharing it will only dilute its power to make you feel peaceful and whole.

*I go to my secret place where I
learn to enjoy solitude and
communion.*

# DAY 220

*Mad at C. J. Walker.*

From this day forward, we hereby decree: good hair no longer means long, straight hair. Enough. Black women are still singing the "Bad Hair Blues":

> He said he loved me,
> but still I ain't happy
> I got me a weave
> but underneath, it's still very nappy
> I got the bad hair bluesss . . .

We've got to get over this thing about hating our hair. Why couldn't Madam C. J. Walker have discovered a hairstyling method that enhanced the natural beauty of our hair? Here's the new definition of bad hair: lifeless, greasy, burned out, dirty, and split ends. Did you see the word *nappy* in there anywhere? No. Nappy no longer means bad. Good hair is clean, trimmed, conditioned, and as close to virgin as possible. Your hair is your crown. Wear it proudly.

*Good hair is healthy hair, and I've got good hair. (Chant this throughout the day as you run your fingers through your lustrous mane.)*

# DAY 221

*"Girl, please, there ain't no conspiracy to market death to the Black community. You're paranoid."*

You're right. There are *many* conspiracies to market death to the Black community, and some of the brightest, most creative Black advertising professionals have been hired to make cigarettes and alcohol look exciting. One tobacco company made a cigarette just for us, and would have been successful, too, had not a Dr. Louis Sullivan called the company to task for its unethical behavior. Black actors, singers, and rappers are being used to sell the particularly lethal 40-ounce malt liquor. The use of rappers is truly satanic, for they appeal to young people. No one likes to admit they're affected by external manipulation, so the idea of a conspiracy is often the butt of jokes. Laugh if you will, while research studies continue to document the rise in alcohol and drug abuse among adults and young people. The good news is, we can resist. We don't have to engage in dangerous behaviors. The choice is ours. Good health begins with a simple decision.

*It's time for the Sleeping Giant to awaken. I refuse to buy anything that's bad for me.*

# DAY 222

*Music is powerful. Music is magical.*

If you feel yourself dragging during your workout, use inspirational music with a beat to pep you up. Modern gospel music is great for this purpose. Your workouts will be transformed into prayer and praise sessions for the Creator. You won't get tired. To the contrary. Stretch your arms high, and reach toward the heavens. Sing, shout, and praise as you move. As you power walk, imagine your Beloved walking right next to you. You'll actually find yourself looking forward to your next workout.

*My workouts are energized with magical, inspired music.*

# DAY 223

*"Girl, I don't feel like cooking tonight."*

When we eat out, we lose control over the food we eat. You need to take control for the sake of your health. Start by asking the waiter questions. What kind of oil have these fries been cooked in? Lard is the wrong answer. Don't let the chef toss your salad; ask for the dressing on the side. Make sure your meats are well done, and by all means, keep a glass of water by your plate at all times. If you must have dessert, quick, cut your serving in half. Keep one-half for yourself, and give the other half back to the waiter.

*I will try to cook more.*

# DAY 224

*Reprioritize your priorities.*

Has your health and fitness program taken a back seat to all the other issues and responsibilities in your life? Has it gotten lost in the life shuffle? You've got to make it a priority. If you're not healthy, you won't be able to handle your load of responsibilities. If you're not fit, you won't have the energy to perform. Health and fitness must take the front seat. It can no longer be a side issue, one that you'll get around to if you get the time. Now's the time.

*Health and fitness is on the top of my "to do" list.*

# DAY 225

*The sad truth is that . . . afflictions, and their unbelievable increase, are the result of the American habit of putting "garbage" in their stomach instead of in the disposal.*
—DICK GREGORY[23]

Comedian turned civil rights activist turned health guru Dick Gregory must assume his rightful place in this book that seeks, above all, the mental, spiritual, physical, and emotional healing of Black women in America. Some might consider Gregory's conspiracy theories to be as extreme as his vegetarian/fasting lifestyle. But no one can deny his commitment to Black health. He believes that most diseases and ailments—"swollen ankles, rheumatism, ulcers, sinus trouble, eye trouble, mental illness, gallstones, prostate gland trouble, hemorrhoids, heart trouble, liver trouble, kidney trouble, overweight, underweight, anemia, bad feet, headaches, short breath, can't sleep or can't wake up, no energy, 'tired' blood"— are all the results of bad eating habits. These are wholly preventable evils, which means we have it within our power to take control of our lives today.

*I have the information, and I'm going to start making the right decisions.*

# DAY 226

*The eating is easy in the summertime.*

Summertime is the time for family reunions, picnics, and barbecues. What these events have in common are food, food, and more food. Black folks love to party, especially when there's free food on the table. While it's great to reestablish old ties, it's another thing to "just say no" to the ribs, potato salad, and bean pie staring you in the face. Have you ever passed on going to the church picnic because you knew you'd never be able to refuse the food? Wait a minute! You don't have to refuse the foods you love. Just exercise moderation. Take long, passionate minutes eating that rib or two (not a slab). Take a couple of teaspoons of potato salad—no more. Eat *slowly,* let the food settle. Now, *go play.* That's right. Don't sit on the picnic bench, sucking your teeth and gossiping. Go play some touch football, piggy, or volleyball with the kids. *Have fun.*

*I won't pig out at the party. I can handle it.*

*Don't quit!*

Not now, not when you've been doing so well. Look, exercising is not just about looking good, it's about feeling good. It's about health. Seems like every day a new study comes out testifying to the benefits of exercise. It builds bone density, which can prevent osteoporosis. Aerobic exercise helps to heal the heart. Exercise unleashes endorphins in the brain. Exercise may help in the battle against breast cancer. Exercise helps diabetics and asthmatics keep their ailments under control. Exercise strengthens the muscles that support arthritic joints. Exercise makes you feel good.

*I can't stop now. Exercise is one of the ways I say "I love you" to my body.*

# DAY 228

*I love my tummy.*

Those fashion models sure make life difficult for us real women, don't they? The ideal of the rippling stomach (no stretch marks) is a difficult one to attain, especially if you've had a baby or two. Is it really necessary to have a "perfect" stomach? The ideal should be health and strength. The stronger your stomach muscles, the less the pressure on your back. Big bellies throw body alignment off, which puts stress on the lower back muscles. Sit-ups alone won't strengthen and tone stomach muscles. In fact, you can do a thousand sit-ups a day, but if you're overweight, you'll probably still have a protruding stomach. The high price tag of tummy tucks often makes cosmetic surgery not an option. A combination of exercise, spot toning, and a low-fat (25 grams a day) eating program is your best bet.

*Even though sit-ups aren't the most fun thing I do during the day, it's one of the best things I do for my body.*

# DAY 229

*Boost your immune system.*

The immune system was on everyone's lips when AIDS first made its evil presence known in the world. In a healthy person, bad (vs. good) bacteria, viruses, and parasites are regularly repelled by white blood cells that are produced by the thymus, lymph nodes, spleen, and bone marrow. The complete breakdown of the immune system leaves the body vulnerable to a whole host of diseases, including cancers, pneumonia, and tuberculosis, among others. In this day and age, don't even think about having unprotected sex. For most of us, our concern about the immune system involves making sure that we commit to a program of healthy eating and exercise. Take those vitamin Cs to ward off colds and flu. Some even believe vitamin C helps to prevent cancer. Stress-relief techniques, such as sitting in nature, prayer and meditation, and listening to music, also help to strengthen your body's fortress against disease and sickness. Get plenty of rest and if, heaven forbid, you get sick, take as much time as you need to recuperate.

*My resistance to disease and sickness is enhanced through my health and fitness program.*

# DAY 230

*Don't be a sissy.*

Weights are for women too! Women often run from weight training, scared that they're going to look like Mr. T. Unless you're into professional body building, there's slim chance of you bulking up. In fact, adding a weight training component to your exercise program can do great things for your body, from building bone density to toning flab. Muscles are expert at burning fat; flab is even better at storing it. You want muscles. You don't have to invest in a health club membership or in fancy equipment. Dumbbells will do just fine. Lots of repetitions using light 3- to 5-pound weights (vs. heavy weights with low repetitions) will create the toned body we're all lusting for.

*I'm no sissy. Lifting weights makes me feel confident and strong. I can take on the world!*

# DAY 231

*Let's make health and fitness a Black thang.*

Our culture is so creative and wonderful. Our dress, walk, talk, dances, foods, music, and styles of worship— our ways are admired and studied throughout the world. Unfortunately, some negatives have crept in and, like a cancer, they are growing wild. We can check them now. Let's build on our strengths to create a new cultural ethos of health and sanity. Let's sing about it and dance to it. Let's braid health, and wrap kente cloth around that.

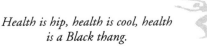

*Health is hip, health is cool, health is a Black thang.*

# DAY 232

*"Girl, I'm thinking about getting me some home training."*

Home training needs to be redefined. In the old days, it meant the manners your mama taught you. As we approach the new millennium, home training must take on a new connotation for a new race of healthy people. The new home training is about getting fit at home when your schedule does not permit a trip to the health club or the park. Home training permits no excuses. Work out at home to videotapes, TV exercise shows, or to your favorite music.

*My home training is about a healthy, no-excuses approach to life.*

# DAY 233

*Stuff happens.*

Sure it does, but why does it have to happen all at once? It rains, the tire gets a flat, and you just had your hair done. That's just the kind of stress that makes you feel justified in reaching for a brownie. Hold it. That's lame, and you know it. Stuff is going to happen, and you can't plan for every eventuality. All you can do sometimes is go with the flow and hang on tight for the ride. It'll calm down in a minute.

*I have within me the power to change myself and my life. I have the serenity to accept the things outside my world that I cannot change.*

# DAY 234

*There's good news and bad news about the yo-yo.*

(No, the yo-yo's not the latest dance.) The good news is that the latest crop of researchers to study yo-yo dieting have discovered that losing and gaining weight over and over has no real effect on your future ability to lose weight. The bad news is, losing and gaining weight over and over wreaks havoc on your self-worth. The vicious dieting cycle, the constant feelings of failure, can mess with your belief in your ability to stick to a health and fitness program. Don't start again until you're really ready to handle the commitment. A promise to self is a sacred bond and should not be treated lightly. Until you're ready to commit, do little things, like walking more and drinking a glass more of water a day. And when you're ready, the resolve will be there.

*No more yo-yo dieting. It's just not worth it. I'm keeping this promise to myself.*

# DAY 235

*The best motivation is internal.*

Sometimes it's hard to feel motivated. We're so conditioned to respond to the push from others that we forget about our innate ability to motivate ourselves. This is a gift and a power. Our baby steps in self-motivation are usually linked to events, such as class reunions or weddings. Maturity develops when we realize that motivation must grow during the process of maintaining a health and fitness lifestyle. This is harder, but ultimately more rewarding and long-lasting.

*Every day I am fired up about my ability and efforts to recreate my body.*

# DAY 236

*Once you go low-fat, it's hard to go back.*

**WARNING:** If you've been consistently eating low-fat foods over an extended period of time, high-fat, greasy foods may be hazardous to your health. The temptations may be strong at parties and picnics to pig out, but resist. You'll end up with a hangover in the morning—nausea, dizzy spells, the whole nine yards. Just be careful. Nibble here and there if you must. Sneak in a slice of your own healthy version of sweet potato pie. If you're worried about offending your host (Black cooks can carry on if you're not gorging yourself on their food), tell her you're allergic to grease.

*My resolve is strong, even in the midst of temptation.*

# DAY 237

*Climb up that mountain, Black women.*

Want firm, sexy love thighs and calves that just beg for a miniskirt? Here's the cheapest piece of exercise equipment yet: climb your behind up the stairs. The exercise industry has made a fortune on something called a Step, which is just a piece of block that you dance up and down on. Save your money for that outfit you've had your eye on. Climbing stairs are great for toning the legs, and as an aerobic exercise, there are few better for strengthening the heart. If there are stairs at work, don't take the elevator—climb. Don't just go for the ride—climb up the escalator. Are there bleachers at your neighborhood park? Climb the steps!

*I'm climbing everyday for firm,*
*beautiful legs and a healthy heart.*

# DAY 238

*"Girl, I just don't know if I can go on."*

Burnout is the malaise of our age. We have so much to do, and so little time. If you've been making a lot of mistakes lately, or if you've been feeling weepy, disoriented, and forgetful, maybe it's time for a break. Just stop. You say you can't? You've got too much to do? Sister, something's got to give, and we don't want it to be your health, now do we? If you don't stop, your wise body will eventually shut down for you. Don't let yourself get sick, instead chill. Send the kids to a relative, take a mental health day at work, and get away if you can. Or stay home and sleep the day away. Don't clean, and most importantly, don't talk to anyone; take the phone off the hook. Or go to your favorite spot in nature and just be quiet and still. Tomorrow you'll be refreshed and ready to handle anything.

*I give myself permission to take
care of my own needs today.*

# DAY 239

*Make big bucks in the exercise industry.*

Since access to quality health care and personal prevention programs are often directly connected to how much money you have, here's a way to make more money so you can buy a personal chef, a personal trainer, an expensive health club membership, a masseuse, and a cosmetic surgeon. Invent an exercise machine. It doesn't have to be anything fancy; in fact, the simpler, the crazier, the better. Look at all the gadgets that are making folks millions of dollars: steps, slides (with special shoes), winglike thigh devices, tummy tuckers, sweat belts, sneakers with flashing lights and pumps—the sky's the limit.

*I get the point. I don't have to heed the hype. All I need are my sweats, my gym shoes, and some wide open spaces.*

# DAY 240

*Menstruation: curse, blessing, or necessary nuisance?*

Ancient women believed that menstruation was a special time of heightened awareness and sensitivity, so they isolated themselves from the tribe and did women's spiritual work. Today we have no such luxury. Period or no, we have to continue to work at home or at the job. To get through the moon time, we take pain pills, and we scream and holler. Personal issues that we managed to hold at bay suddenly gush to the surface like a geyser, forcing us to deal with them. Let's take our cue from those wise ancient women. Although realistically we can't go live in a hut for a week every month, we can insist on taking meditation time for ourselves. This cleansing time is as much for our emotions and spirit as it is for our bodies.

*My period is not a curse; it is a blessing in disguise.*

# DAY 241

*"No more cloudy days. I need some sun!"*

Black women need the sun. We look so good in the sun, with the rays bouncing off our tan, brown, and black skins. Unfortunately, many of us can only access the sun's healing rays on the weekends. By the time we get off work, the sun's already beginning to set in the west. If a job threatens to separate you from this rich source of vitamin D and inspiration, make sure you get out during lunchtime. Don't let a heavy workload rob you of the sun's warm caress. There's nothing like the feeling of sun on our skin. We've been counseled against sunbathing, and it's true that even too much of a good thing can be bad for you; luckily sunblock can protect the skin from the sun's more harmful ultraviolet rays. But understand, as people of the sun, we must, for health and sanity, get our daily dose.

*Warm sunny rays bathe my body and soothe my nerves. I'll make time for the sun.*

# DAY 242

*Self-love means being unafraid of solitude.*

Being alone with our thoughts can be unnerving, which is why we tend to surround ourselves with people, activity, and noise. Learning to love the silence is a courageous undertaking, and well worth the effort. In solitude, there's no one to justify us, reinforce us, or motivate us but ourselves. Solitude challenges us to rely on our inner resources. Don't run from the opportunity to spend quality time with yourself. Embrace solitude with open arms.

*I welcome the peace of solitude and
the learning opportunities it offers.*

# DAY 243

*Let's not confuse our outer shells with our inner selves.*

What makes you special? Does it have anything to do with your body, or does it have to do with who you are inside? Does the uniqueness of your secret self lie in the fact that your essence is a nurturing one? Is your secret your rolling hips of thunder, or is it the sassy spark that animates them? Do men simply love your shapely legs, or the sturdiness within you that roots them in Mama Earth? Lest we confuse the outer shell with the inner woman, never doubt that it is your essence that shapes your physical body. All the makeup in the world cannot hide an ugly soul. And we all know women who, though not "classically" beautiful, glow from within. They make us feel good just being around them, and we begin to see their true beauty. Your thoughts, emotions, and values help to mold what your body eventually becomes.

*I am an amazingly beautiful
woman, inside and out.*

# DAY 244

*Have you been putting your life on hold?*

Many women pass on social events because they're just too embarrassed to be seen the "way they are." They could be a mere five pounds to a hundred pounds overweight, it doesn't matter. How many of us have missed our tenth high school reunion because we were ashamed of how we looked? Maybe you've had a baby or two, or maybe not, but you no longer look like sweet sixteen. You've put on a few extra pounds, or maybe over the years gravity has redistributed the same pounds differently. But, guess what—everyone is feeling the ravages of time. Men go bald and grow love handles and beer bellies. And we all begin to gray sooner or later. Waistlines have thickened because we've slowed down. For too many of us, stressful, sedentary jobs have replaced our once active lifestyles. The moral of this story? No one will be looking sweet sixteen at the reunion. The problem lies not in how time has treated us, but in how we think about ourselves.

*With all that said and done, I ain't going down without a fight!*

# DAY 245

*If it seems too good to be true, it probably is.*

Crash diets, pills, sauna suits, cellulite cream, and exercise contraptions have all been hyped as the ultimate miracle products, promising weight loss and model bodies. So we spend our hard-earned dollars on all manner of junk. We might even lose a pound or two, but inevitably we'll gain it back, plus some—just ask Oprah. The hardest lesson to accept in the weight-loss war is that the miracles are far and few in between. The majority of us must resign ourselves to the fact that it will take hard work and discipline to achieve our health and fitness goals. The good news is, it can be done! We can do it! Contrary to what the scientific community would have us believe, fat recidivism is not inevitable. While the success stories may be in the minority, those are the ones we must look to for guidance, hope, and inspiration.

*I'm not looking for a quick fix. I'm in this for the long haul.*

# DAY 246

*Are you holding a grudge against anyone?*

"I'll forgive, but I'll never forget." How many times have you said that about someone who hurt you? If you haven't forgotten, you're still holding on to the past. Learn the lesson from the pain, then drop it. Old hurts sometimes feel like old luggage: you can never get rid of them. But you've got to. Grudges are weights that drag you down. One grudge probably weighs the physical equivalent of a ton of fat, maybe two, maybe ten. The point is, grudges are extremely heavy burdens to carry around, and they could be manifesting themselves as extra weight, even sickness, on your body.

*No slight is worth sacrificing my health and sanity. I let go of all old grudges.*

*Self-consciousness is you looking back at yourself—and not liking what you see.*

When you look in the mirror, how do you feel? In a glance, do you see and react in disgust to your less-than-perfect body? Do you take in the slumped shoulders, the double chin, the sagging breasts, the protruding stomach, the rippling thighs? If you've been struggling with body issues for a long time, you have probably reached the level of extreme self-consciousness—and self-hatred. You just don't feel comfortable in your body. Adding to this feeling is the perception that you're drowning in a sea of skinny people. Everywhere you go, happy thin people seem to be enjoying life, while you seem destined to be a spectator forever. Over the years your self-consciousness builds into a crescendo, an obsession. Layer upon layer of self-loathing. Hold it! You've got to get a grip. It's true that American society is pathological about its fears of physical differences—including heaviness (not to mention our African features). But that doesn't mean we have to accept their ideals of beauty. It comes down to this: we must love and accept ourselves, and we must be supportive of each other.

*When I look in the mirror, I like what I see.*

# DAY 248

*Eating day-old bread is like settling for a rabbit coat when you really wanted a mink.*

Without a doubt, our history of slavery, poverty, and despair in America has made its devastating impact on our state of mind and physical health. Even though some of us have managed to achieve a modicum of success, we all have to struggle against the poverty mentality. The poverty mentality has us settling for poor quality food, which, of course, barely satisfies our physical need for nourishment, much less our sensual need for taste. It's strange, but the more you eat the stale food often sold in our neighborhood grocery stores, the more you want and the less you're satisfied. The higher the food quality, the less you'll feel the need to eat. Even if you have to go out of your way, buy only the freshest fruits, vegetables, meat, and poultry. Cost should not be an issue. In fact, the high-quality foods sold in the suburbs are often cheaper than the poor excuse for food that's sold in our communities.

*I'll buy and eat the freshest foods because I'm worth it.*

# DAY 249

*The longest journey begins with a single step.*

Little by little, create a new lifestyle that will support your health and fitness goals. You might find yourself changing aspects of your life that appear to have no tangible connection to losing weight or toning muscles. Say you've gotten the urge to start buying flowers for your home. How do flowers tie in to losing weight? If flowers make you feel happy, if just looking at flowers help heal your mind and soul, you'll feel more motivated to engage in positive life-changing activities, like exercise. It's just that simple. Take just one single step, and then another and another. You'll be laying the foundation, piece by piece, for a new healthy life.

*Everything I do, no matter how seemingly insignificant, creates a new mindset of health and fitness within me.*

# DAY 250

*"Girl, I just bought a book about losing weight. I want to lose fifty pounds."*

Does buying a diet thing cause weight loss? Judging from the billions of dollars we've been pouring into the diet industry, we must believe that the act of writing checks and pulling plastic and cash out of our wallets burns calories. We buy everything from aromatherapy smelling tubes to wacky exercise equipment to books and tapes to memberships in weight-loss clubs. Look, apart from buying this wonderful book for all your sisterfriends (smile), don't spend another dime. Some things in life really are free, like exercise, prayer, and meditation. Fresh quality food should cost no more than the junk food you've been buying. Let's invest the money we save into our own communities to build economic strength so that all of our people will have access to quality products and services, including health care.

*Advertising hype and my own desperation have no effect whatsoever on my purchasing decisions. Losing weight will take perseverance and discipline, and I'm more than equal to the task.*

# DAY 251

*God is great, God is good. Let us thank Her for our food. Amen.*
—CHILDREN'S MEALTIME PRAYER

Let's get back to blessing our food before the first bite, even if it's only a snack. Prayer puts us into a receptive frame of mind. Prayer opens our bodies to receiving the vitamins and nutrients that the food offers us. And don't pray the same old tired prayer that you've long since lost the meaning and power of. Pray creatively and carefully. Pray that an ailing body part be healed by the food. Pray that the food actually raises your sluggish metabolism. Now believe, and believe with all your heart that this food will do a good work within your body.

*I am thankful for this food that is rich in nutrients and exquisite in taste.*

# DAY 252

*What's that smell?*

Lately, there's been a lot of excited talk about a "new age" healing technology called aromatherapy that may have some meaningful application to weight-loss efforts. People who participated in research studies did lose weight by whiffing, without consciously reducing calories or even exercising. Apparently, smelling scents like strawberries or baked bread actually triggers the satisfaction mechanism in our brains, which, theoretically, prevents overeating. Other scents, like baby powder, can soothe last nerves.[24] Who knows? It could work. Stranger things have happened.

*There have been times when unusual ideas have made a positive impact on my life. This could be one of those times.*

# DAY 253

*Are you on automatic?*

Eating should be a major production. You should be aware of every delicious morsel that enters your mouth. Unfortunately, those of us who are compulsive overeaters often miss out on the pleasure of eating because the robotic process of shoveling takes over. Scoop up the food, shovel it in. By the time your plate is clean, not only have you forgotten what you just ate, you've misplaced the capacity to taste. So you go for seconds and thirds because you're never satisfied. Let's take a Zen-like approach to eating. Be aware of every bite. Notice tastes and textures. As you practice this eating meditation, you'll become aware of an amazing thing: satisfaction. Staying awake during eating can help in weight loss as you become more aware of true hunger levels. Imagine the freedom of actually being able to put your fork down once satisfaction has been recognized.

*I am awake, I am conscious, I am aware. I will not lapse into the deep sleep of robotic eating.*

*Pissed-off babies grow up to be pissed-off adults.*
—DR. CARL BELL, PSYCHOLOGIST

Child abuse is a public health disgrace of increasing concern, and Black mothers have become a favorite target of news programs and talk shows. Black mothers (and fathers indirectly) are being maligned in the media as abusive to children, perpetrating every sort of terrorism. To set the record straight, most Black mothers are doing their job, and doing it well despite the lack of societal, community, and even familial support. But the truth be told, we know that the problem is increasing, and it coincides with the escalation of crack-cocaine addiction, poverty, and teen pregnancy in our community. Needless to say, there are no easy answers. We are all responsible, collectively and individually, for the mental and physical health of our children.

*It's time to regroup for the health and safety of our children, families, and communities.*

# DAY 255

*Once upon a time . . .*

. . . there was a woman named Evelyn. For years, she had tried to lose weight, and was sometimes even successful. Then some tragedy would strike, usually involving a man, and she'd fall off the wagon. "I'm only a woman," she'd say to her friends, smiling through her tears, as she ate ice cream straight out of the tub. As the years went by, Evelyn grew bigger and bigger. Her self-worth was nonexistent and she became near suicidal. One Saturday evening, as she sat at home alone watching TV and gorging on bean pie and ice cream, she suddenly felt sick to her stomach. She made it to the bathroom just in time. She felt as sick as an alley drunk, and knew she had hit rock bottom. For the first time in years, the tears flowed like a cleansing rain, and she began to remember. Memories flashed like snapshots in her mind—painful, embarrassing memories. She called her pastor, and they talked for hours. The first step in Evelyn's healing was the most painful, but she took it. She made that phone call. Without the first step, the healing cannot happen.

*Trying to lose weight without addressing underlying issues, whatever they may be, is a setup for failure.*

# DAY 256

*Homemade exercise equipment—a newborn baby.*

Infants can make for some of the sweetest, most effective homemade progressive resistance equipment. As they grow, your muscles will become increasingly challenged, which results in strength and tone. To begin this googoo gaga weight-training program, simply find a newborn baby. Lie down, back on the floor, knees up to relieve pressure on the back. Hold the baby securely around its waist and lift it high into the air. Tightening your chest muscles, lower the baby gradually. Repeat 15 times. (Do not do this exercise immediately following the kid's dinner.) For aerobic conditioning, carry the baby in a front or back pouch as you take your daily walk. Not only will the extra weight strengthen your heart's pumping action and burn fat, you and the baby will bond for a lifetime.

*Who says babies are cheap exercise equipment? College alone will cost $100,000!*

# DAY 257

*Got the blues?*

Color affects our moods in subtle, often subconscious ways. Wearing red clothes can give us energy. Blue rooms can calm us down, or even depress us. If you're feeling stressed, you'll probably not want to eat in a red room or on brightly colored plates. Maybe you shouldn't wear pastel sweats if you've been dragging on your walk. Wear bright, bold colors to psyche yourself up. Many books have been written on how colors influence human emotion and intellect, but don't depend on what other people say. Meditate on a variety of colors to understand your own responses. Be mindful of how colors affect your eating and workout sessions.

*Color me calm. Color me passionate. Color me disciplined. Color me healthy.*

# DAY 258

*Keep on moving. Don't stop!*

There's nothing like disappointment in self to obliterate all traces of motivation and a positive spirit. But remember when you were a girl jumping double-dutch?
There were times when you missed, but that didn't stop
you. As soon as your turn came around, you got right
back into the game. Stop digging your mashed potatoes!
All this fretting about disappointment and failure will
get you nowhere. The only way to get back on your program is to get back on your program.

*Everyone backslides, but I refuse to
allow setbacks to detour me from
the pursuit of my health and
fitness goals.*

# DAY 259

*The secret of Oprah's success: If at first you don't succeed, try, try again.*

At least when *you* blow it your setbacks aren't publicized on national TV. Weight for women is such a sensitive issue. Like her or not, you've got to give it to Oprah Winfrey. She faced the cameras day in and day out, regardless of her size. Oprah also dispelled a myth that has been promoted for years by so-called diet experts—that yo-yo dieting ultimately reduces the effectiveness of the body to lose weight. Not true, thank God! Oprah's success shows us that we can overcome both the low self-worth that comes from yo-yoing and eliminate the unwanted pounds.

*If Oprah can do it, so can I. I'll be my own chef and personal trainer. I can do this.*

# DAY 260

*Why do you want to lose weight?*

Unfortunately, American society promotes a good thing like loss of excess weight for all the wrong reasons. Sure, you may look better in your clothes after the loss of a few pounds, but that's only a side benefit. The real deal about weight loss should be health and prevention. If you're basically a healthy person, prevention may seem like a vague reason to embark on a wellness program, but consider this: researchers are beginning to admit that bad diet and stress cause most major illnesses and many diseases. Exercise in your younger years can help prevent old age ailments like osteoporosis. Depression can be greatly alleviated, if not cured, by exercise. A thin body should never be your goal. Aim for health and fitness.

*I know I want to be thinner, but that's beside the point—I'm going for 100 percent perfect health.*

# DAY 261

*What's the most lived-in room in the house?*

The kitchen! In fact, the kitchen should be renamed the living room. While the living rooms in most Black homes stand as immaculate plastic museums, our kitchens virtually sing with smells and talk. We press hair there and we cook collards, onions, and chocolate cakes there. We eat there and we share there. The kitchen is the heart of our homes. Stock it well with non-stick cooking pans, a wok, a blender, and healthy fresh foods and herbs.

*My well-stocked kitchen is a reflection of my new healthy lifestyle.*

# DAY 262

*Desperate women do desperate things.*

Is your biological clock ticking? Are you manless or jobless? Still can't shed those extra pounds? Desperation drives many a smart Black woman to commit acts that would, under normal circumstances, be considered insane. Crash dieting and promiscuous, unprotected sex are the acts of a desperate woman. Don't give in to those urgent, out-of-control feelings. Take a deep breath, calm down, and learn to draw strength, patience, and wisdom from within. Acts committed under the screaming and yelling of desperate emotions seldom lead to anything positive.

*I will learn patience and wait for
the things I desire. I will persevere.*

# DAY 263

*You are a queen.*

The lie handed down to us from European and African monarchies is that royalty is inherited, and that for some really weird reason, being born into a particular family gives you certain privileges. We've been taught that we can't be queens unless we are born into the "right" family. Wrong! Queenship is your divine right. You assume the queenship through your divine inheritance. You are God's daughter, an earthly queen. America does not have a monarchy, but the idea of royal inheritance is just as strong here as it is in Britain or was in ancient Egypt. It is all about power and control. Assume your rightful position as a beautiful Black queen in your home, on your job, in your church, mosque, or temple, and in your community. Rule *yourself* with class, wisdom, and patience. You are worthy of respect and love, and have earned the right to be called Queen.

*From princess to queen, I have learned to rule wisely over my emotions, mind, and body.*

# DAY 264

*The void is the scary deep place where your innermost desires reside.*

People can have high self-worth but still have a void in their lives. The desire to have a baby, to be married, to go back to school, to have a slimmer body—anything that you deeply desire that has eluded you, maybe for years, is the unrealized desire that festers in the void. If they are not dealt with, voids will create vulnerability to all kinds of influences. We tend to want to run away from voids because they are so painful; they sap our energy. Black holes in space are powerful because they suck in all the light; our personal voids suck in our energy. All of our attention focuses on desires that still lie in the realm of dreams. The only way to make peace with the void is to talk right into it. We must have the courage to ask ourselves, "Why have I not yet manifested this desire? What purpose does this longing serve?"

*Today I make peace with my soul's deepest longing. Either I will let it go, once and for all, or I will take steps toward its fulfillment.*

# DAY 265

*Do you rise up singing or boohooing?*

The way you wake up can set the tone for the entire day. If you wake up grumbling about having to get up, or if you're hungover from last night, or if you're achy and sore from sleeping on a bad mattress, you'll probably find yourself struggling to get through the day. Before you get up to do anything, take a few deep breaths and pray. Be thankful for your life and this new day to start fresh. Bless the day's upcoming tasks. Then stretch like a cat, stretch all the kinks out. Drink a tall glass of water or juice, and eat a power-packed breakfast. You'll be surprised how much more smoothly your day will flow.

*With the rising sun, my energy and
my spirits soar.*

# DAY 266

*"Girl, I got to get me some sleep."*

Remember when as a little girl you used to fight sleep? You probably thought you would miss out on something important if you went to sleep. What's bedtime been like for you lately? Have you had trouble sleeping, or do you sleep so hard you wake up with a headache? Have you been getting enough sleep? Bedtime is so important. A few years ago, some demented scientists deprived cats of sleep to see how they'd act. Specifically, the poor creatures were not allowed to experience REM (rapid eye movement), that deep part of sleep in which dreams occur. How did they think they'd act? They went berserk. You will too if you don't get your eight hours.

*Now I lay me down to sleep . . .*

# DAY 267

*Self-love means letting go of restrictions and inhibitions.*

Freedom! That's a concept that we Black women need to really absorb deep into our souls. Too many of us have resorted to alcohol and drugs in order to feel free. That's when we let down the barriers to conservative behavior and shoo away all our tiresome inhibitions. Even though we might keep her hidden, we all have a wild and crazy woman who wants to come out and play. If we don't let her out occasionally, she'll bust loose and wreak havoc in our lives. If we let her out responsibly, our lives will be enhanced and we'll have much more fun. If your wild woman wants palm trees painted on her fingernails, do it! If she wants to swing in the park with the kids, let her out. If she wants an occasional slice of bean pie, let her have it.

*I love the wild, untamed part of me.*

# DAY 268

*Subtraction = Deprivation*

When trying to lose weight, don't subtract. Don't think in terms of all the greasy or sweet foods you're going to be giving up. Think of all the delicious, healthy foods you're going to be adding to your eating program. It's the new math, and a new way of thinking about health. Why should health and fitness be yet another chore in the day to get through? Instead, eating and exercising should be pleasurable time-outs during the day. Add homemade honey lemonade with mint, fresh fruit desserts, and low-fat vegetable casseroles. Add dancing. There's no reason on earth why your life should be miserable. Add spice. Add fun.

*I'm not taking away anything by adding the health factor to my life.*

# DAY 269

*Do you fear intimacy?*

Closeness can be threatening. As you get closer to another person, the real you is revealed. The more exposed you are, the more vulnerable you are. We Black women have millions of stories to tell about love gone bad, and we've got plenty of scars to show. The natural reaction is to want to protect yourself from future pain. Seldom are fear and related issues resolved by building walls around our hearts, engaging in one-night stands, overeating, or becoming workaholics. These are all strategies to avoid dealing with the main problem: fear of intimacy. And for a time they may appear to work. In the long run, however, they will prove a barrier to the union we want. Before jumping into a sexual relationship, embark on a program to develop yourself—in health and fitness, education, career, and spiritual development.

*I will learn to trust again.*
*I will demystify men. I will get to*
*know them as friends and humans*
*first before rushing into sex.*

# DAY 270

*Do you bore even yourself?*

Has your life become one big yawn? No wonder we eat too much sometimes. Flavors provide at least some stimulation in an otherwise humdrum existence. But ask yourself this question: What's the point of being so bored that mealtime is the most exciting event of the day? It's time for a change. Look at your life honestly. There's something that you want to do. What's holding you back? Fear? A title of a book says *Feel the Fear and Do It Anyway.* That's what it comes down to, having the courage to step into unknown territory and knowing that the entire universe is there to catch you. Whether its getting married or divorced, taking a new job, or moving to a new country, you can't deny your heart's longing. The denial will only cause stress, which is not good for your health, our primary concern.

*I'm going to take risks for a
magnificent life.*

# DAY 271

*What are you thinking?*

Thousands of thoughts rush through our minds during the course of a day. Think of your mental dialogue as a gigantic stream. Every time you think a negative thought, a toxin drips into your bloodstream. Drip by drip, your thoughts can tangibly affect how healthy or how sick you are. Each drop can be a drop of poison or a drop of life. Changing your thoughts from negative to positive can be difficult, but definitely not impossible. All it takes is a decision. And a thought.

*The more positive my thoughts, the healthier my body.*

# DAY 272

*Are you a cosmic or a cosmetic beauty?*

One of the reasons why we tend to be so susceptible to the hype of the image industry is because we define beauty according to external standards, and European ones at that. Cosmetic beauties really know how to apply that makeup. They have their nails and hair done every week, but don't have a clue as to who they are inside, or who they are in the universal scheme of things. A cosmic beauty is a Black woman who knows that external beauty is merely a function of internal beauty, and that the more the Spirit is allowed to shine, the less cosmetics ultimately matter.

*I am a cosmic beauty.*
*I enter the holy realm*
*of personal power, health,*
*and beauty.*

*Sexism is irrelevant.*

There's a victim mentality prevalent among women today that threatens to sap our power. Black women are batted about by so many "isms," we run a real risk of resorting to blaming others for the decisions we make. Feminists love to blame men for everything, which is so much easier than assuming responsibility for self. Yes, there's abuse, violence, and more, but victim mathematics doesn't necessarily compute. There may have been sexual abuse in childhood, but that does not have to lead to eating disorders. We still have the power of decision, and we can decide to get help. As adult women, we must choose mental health over self-pity and self-destructive behaviors.

*I will change my whole life if I have to. I'll get help. I will be healed.*

# DAY 274

*Dare to know you're beautiful.*

We who have experienced the deep, deep psychic pain of being deemed by society as not beautiful must draw on the strength and creativity of our foremamas. They knew how to create something out of nothing, and we cannot afford to be any less resourceful. Begin by realizing that you are beauty personified. Dare to see the beauty of your so-called imperfections. Stretch marks are now your stripes of honor. Cellulite contains valuable information about your past. Broad shoulders bear the burdens of the world. Heavy low-lying breasts nurture men, women, and children. Your body is not ugly. It is a monument to your internal and external beauty. It is a library of stored information about yourself, your thoughts, feelings, and past experiences. Think on these things and now, when you look at yourself in the mirror, give yourself a wink and a smile.

*Who is that outrageously gorgeous creature in the mirror? It's me!*

# DAY 275

*Fake food is not the best food.*

All fake foods carry risks and we must wonder, are they really necessary? MSG (monosodium glutamate) and fat and sugar substitutes are fake foods that contain no nutritional value whatsoever. In fact, many have been found to produce side effects, such as dizziness and headaches. And, dieters, studies have shown that in the long run, artificial sweeteners may actually undermine your weight-loss efforts. Dieters tend to eat more high-calorie foods to make up for the lack of calories in, for example, zero-calorie sodas. Rather than putting your health in jeopardy, it would be much wiser to eat foods containing natural ingredients, such as sugar (a little bit), honey, fruit juice sweeteners, and vegetable oils. Just use them responsibly.

*Real food is the best food. I will not allow desperation to get the best of me.*

# DAY 276

*Stressbuster: water falling on your body*

Close your eyes: imagine yourself on a tropical island. It's a warm, sunny day and there's natural beauty all around. Straight ahead is a waterfall. The water is crystal clear and is beckoning to you. Stand in the water. Let its pulsing rhythm wash over your tired muscles. Wouldn't it be great to have access to a waterfall whenever you feel stressed out? You do, and it's in your bathroom. Take a shower. Convert your bathroom into a tropical paradise with plants and scents. You may even want to invest in a massage attachment. It could change your life.

*It feels good to know that I can reduce stress by simply stepping into my bathtub.*

# DAY 277

*Is there such a thing as a family curse?*

In your family, have the sins and weaknesses of the mothers been visited upon the daughters? Mothers teach their daughters by example how to relate to men, how to treat their bodies, and how to cope with stress. Ultimately, you have the final say in how you conduct your life, but you may be unaware of unconscious motivations bequeathed to you by your mother, and her mother, and her mother. And while it's true, our history extends far before slavery, that genocidal institution is responsible for many of the behaviors being played out in our community today. Still, there can be no excuses when it comes to your health. First of all, resolve not to pass on negative behaviors to your daughters and sons. *We could turn it all around in a generation or two!* Then cancel the effects of the curse in your life through your own power of decision.

*Curses are only as powerful as I make them. I accept my power of free will, and cancel any lingering effects of family and cultural curses in my life.*

# DAY 278

*Are you waiting for weight loss before choosing happiness?*

That's right, happiness is a choice. When turmoil is all around you, you must resolve to be happy despite the negatives in your life. Heavy women living in a society that values skinniness often find themselves isolated from the mainstream. Loneliness, depression, and despair become constant companions—unless you decide to choose happiness. Don't wait to lose weight to be happy. Seek out new friendships and love. Give love to receive love.

*I assume responsibility for my emotional healing.*

# DAY 279

*Look at the big picture.*

We each have an entire internal universe to roam in and explore. Black women were created in a wondrous image. We are sparks of divinity. We were blessed with powers, many of which are unknown to us. Our precious lives should be spent exploring our own individual universes. Try not to be consumed by the unimportant things that have no external value. Dig deeply within your soul. You'll be amazed at the reservoirs of beauty and wonder that reside within you.

*In the universal scheme of things, those extra pounds seem pretty trivial.*

# DAY 280

*Who are you trying to please?*

Black women wear many hats—mother, daughter, lover, worker. There's something about being a woman that equates to the need to please. We will often put the needs of others first before taking care of ourselves. In fact, many of us wouldn't know how to please ourselves. So, here's your assignment for the day: figure out a way to make yourself happy. Be pleasing to yourself. Today your primary goal will be to please yourself. What do you want to do today? If you feel guilty about being "selfish," you need to understand that word in a new way. You cannot fulfill your other roles to the best of your ability if you are depleted. Do things that will enhance the health of your body, uplift your spirit, or heal your emotions.

*Today I'm going to take time to please and love myself.*

# DAY 281

*There's a difference between self-esteem and self-worth.*

Self-esteem is the yardstick some psychologists use to measure how we value ourselves. High self-esteem means you feel good about yourself; low self-esteem means you feel a pervading sense of futility about your life. In the past, self-esteem concept had more teeth because it had to be earned; today, it's like a get rich quick scheme. It's like easy money inherited from birth. Here's another, perhaps more revealing definition: self-esteem is our own reflection seen in society's mirror. Self-worth, on the other hand, is earned and driven by the internal cues of integrity and positive values. Self-esteem relates to our external self; self-worth to the inner self. Self-esteem is about cosmetics; self-worth is about character development and our relationship to the cosmos. Self-esteem is not inherently bad; it's just that self-worth is infinitely better.

*My high level of self-worth has been earned through years of meeting challenges head-on. My self-worth empowers my health and fitness efforts.*

# DAY 282

*Are you in touch with your sexuality?*

Touchy subject, but one that must be dealt with as you pursue healing. How you feel about that aspect of your womanhood can inform your eating habits, your relationships, how you dress—anything and everything. Women in general must fight unhealthy media themes linking sexuality to violence, manipulation, social climbing, etc. Media images of Black women do nothing to support a healthy sense of our sexual selves. Music videos depict us as pornographic bitches and hoes. In Hollywood and the news media, we are drug-addicted and completely defeminized. Imagine, though, if we were all fed images of Black women birthing the sun, as in Egyptian mythology. How differently we'd feel about ourselves! How differently others would treat and perceive us! The most damaging thing Western civilization did to our sexuality was to separate it from the sacred. Without a sense of the sacred, our sexuality becomes empty, dirty, or destructive. We open ourselves to all manner of manipulation. Sexuality is more than our sexual organs. It is all of us—and more.

*Creation and my sexuality are one.*

# DAY 283

*Are you a glutton or a compulsive eater?*

In the Bible, Paul talks a lot about the war between the flesh and spirit. He calls gluttony a sin, an evil thing. Today, the scientific community appears to be leaning toward defining obesity as a disease. In fact, the search is on for a gene that may be responsible and the drugs to cure it. Are we sinful gluttons, or are we captive to a biological mechanism out of our control? Or is obesity a little of both? Who knows? Just be aware that much of the treatment heavy people receive is informed by these positions.

*I still have the power to decide what and how much I will eat. I choose health.*

# DAY 284

*Take it off. Take it all off.*

Take off all your clothes and look at yourself in the mirror. How do you feel? Do you turn yourself on, or are you repulsed? Look at your beautiful face, your shoulders, breasts, vagina, and legs. Turn to the side. Look at your stomach and your behind. Oh, Lord! That's a lot of good woman. Now, put on your prettiest lingerie and, just for you, remember your sensuality throughout the day. Eat sexy, healthy foods, and eat them slowly. Take a walk, and swing those African woman hips meaningfully and deliberately.

*I love being a healthy, sensual woman.*

# DAY 285

*If they lied about Columbus . . .*

On Bedloe's Island in New York Harbor stands what's got to be the tallest image of a Caucasian woman on the planet: the Statue of Liberty. She invites the poor, tired, and oppressed to experience the golden streets of America. We know better. More interesting than the rhetoric, however, is the mysterious plot that surrounds Liberty's creation. Rumor has it that Lady Liberty was originally an *African* woman.[25] Just as Michelangelo re-created Jesus in the image of the European man, Lady Liberty was re-created in the image of the American white woman. When the statue was completed in 1883 by Alsatian sculptor Frédéric Auguste Bartholdi, no doubt he was well aware of the hideous institution of American slavery and correctly surmised that the image of an African woman would best depict America's promise of freedom and opportunity. It's unfortunate that he was overruled by the powers that be. How differently would we Black women feel about ourselves had we been raised on that image standing so tall and proud? How differently would we have been treated by others? No matter. Now you know the truth, so let the truth set you free.

*I am freedom personified. I am no longer enslaved by past traumas or negative behaviors.*

*Cry.*

Some aspects of this society's value system are really warped. Take the masculine injunction against tears. The superwoman facade Black women are constantly expected to maintain serves no one, women or men. Society's definition of strength is the absence of emotions, which, of course, only means that the stress has temporarily been pushed down, not healed. Crying heals us. Even the skies cry to cleanse the air and the soil. Tears are our safety valve; without them, all kinds of difficult emotions would remain bottled up inside, causing sickness and suffering. Black women could teach the world to cry, so great has been our collective pain. And with those tears, humanity would begin to heal.

*When I need to cry, I will. I won't stop the flow.*

# DAY 287

*Through childhood traumas
we lose important parts of our Self.*

It's time to reclaim the lost and hidden parts of ourselves. The quest for health is about wholeness. Fragmented, fractured souls will have too many conflicting motivations that can undermine health and fitness efforts. Reclaiming our lost selves is deep, deep emotional and spiritual work. It may involve working through painful memories. *Don't do this alone.* A good therapist can help you push through those experiences you haven't wanted to deal with for years.

*It may take awhile, but I commit
myself to becoming a whole,
healthy woman.*

# DAY 288

*Mother your body.*

Black women are the world's greatest mothers. No other figure in our community is given more respect, love, loyalty, and adoration. She's earned it. Often holding the family together alone, she is strong and resourceful. For those of us who have mothered our own or other people's children, let's give ourselves a pat on the back. Now apply your mothering skills to your health and fitness efforts. Just as we can never give up on our children, we can never give up on ourselves. Just as our children deserve the best we can give them, we are worthy of the freshest foods and quality time to exercise, meditate, and pray.

*I will mother myself. If I don't,
who will?*

# DAY 289

*I love my chin(s).*

It matters not how many chins you have. What matters is how you feel about them. If you don't like what you've got, do something about it. Exercise and beautify those chins. Tilt your head as far back as you can. Open and close your mouth ten times. Feel the stretch of your neck as you close your mouth. Now tilt your head to the right, and open and close your mouth ten times. Repeat on the left side. This time-honored exercise will help firm up the neck and chin area. As for makeup, if you use foundation, please use a color that exactly matches your skin color. Take the time to spread and blend in completely to your chin(s) and neck area.

*My chin(s) adds dignity to my*
*stunning profile.*

# DAY 290

*Take a deep breath.*

Breath is about life. Without it we die. Entire sciences have been created around the breath. According to natural health practitioner Asar Ha-Pi in Chicago, our Egyptian ancestors used breathing in conjunction with yoga-type exercises for vitality and longevity. Deep diaphragm breathing replenishes our energy supply. Simply breathe in deeply for eight counts, filling up your belly with oxygen. Focus on the stomach, not the chest. Repeat two or three times. You should feel revitalized and ready to party.

*I breathe in health, joy, and peace.*
*I exhale poverty, illness, and*
*depression.*

# DAY 291

*Twist like a pretzel.*

Yoga—even if you're not big on the religion, the physical discipline is a healing balm for your body's mechanical problems. The asanas, or postures, develop strength and flexibility. The trick is to do them as honestly as you can, holding them for as many as 10 to 20 seconds at a time, breathing deeply. Deep diaphragm breathing builds much needed reserves of energy. Yoga massages muscles, organs, skeletal, elimination, circulatory, respiratory, and digestive systems. The back and womb postures are especially wonderful for women. The cobra pose (bhujangasana) is a truly heavenly way to knead out the kinks in your back. Lie down on your stomach, with your legs held together straight and tight behind you and your behind muscles clenched. Place your hands on either side of your chest, elbows pointing up in the air. Now, gently, push off the floor. You'll be tempted to use your arms to lift, but don't. Feel the pull in your spine and chest. Remember to breathe, and hold the pose for a slow, easy count of five. Lower, and relax.

*Yoga stretches my limbs and massages my muscles. I feel as limber as a child.*

# DAY 292

*Think like a child.*

Your imagination can be your ally in building your will and motivation. As a child, your imagination was your playmate. As you grew older and became more world-weary and "reality" based, you used your imagination less and less. Don't be dismayed; it may have atrophied some, but, like a muscle, it can be built up again. While you're doing your power walk, imagine a most trusted friend walking with you, encouraging you. As you're lying flat on your back doing hip raises, imagine yourself having sex with some fine specimen of a man. Free your imagination. Let your mind soar.

*In my mind's eye, I can be whomever I want to be. I can imagine myself in whatever situation I desire.*

# DAY 293

*"Girl, I'm not creative."*

Creativity is the great mediator between heaven and earth. It is the spark in us that interprets spiritual perceptions for this earthbound reality. Writers, painters, dancers, and musicians do not have a monopoly on creativity. Black women who love to cook are wonderfully creative. It takes creativity and resourcefulness to raise a child well. We Black people are internationally admired for our ability to be creative in a variety of disciplines, from the sciences to arts and entertainment to sports. Let's rein in our abundant creativity and put it in service to our health and fitness efforts.

*I am a creative woman. New ideas
on staying healthy, fit, and
motivated flow to me in
abundance today.*

# DAY 294

*What time is it?*

Albert Einstein said that time is relative. Although his discovery related to physics, we can understand the relativity of time in a personal way. Think of time as either the Tortoise or the Hare. When you're doing something you hate, time inches along like a Tortoise. When you're doing something you love, time zooms like the Hare. Do you like to exercise? Many of us don't, but we all know we have to. Most of us would prefer Hare time to Tortoise time during workout sessions. Inspirational music with a beat and working out with friends are ways to speed up time. In other words, fun and strong interest are two keys that you can use to make time work on your behalf.

*I know how to stretch or contract
time to serve my purposes.*

# DAY 295

*Real women don't have hot flashes;*
*they have power surges.*

It's time out for accepting victimization as our lot. We
know the forces working against our health—the greasy
food joints, our own inertia, the food industry's billion
dollar advertising budget. But we can withstand all of
that if we simply come into the knowledge of, and begin
to own, our power. For example, we all have known—
or have been—women who couldn't seem to leave a terrible relationship. We beg them, cajole them, try to
shame them, but the sisters seem as if they're trapped
by prison bars. The problem is not the man, no matter
what he's done. The problem is that the woman won't
own the power she has in such abundance. Yes, there's
something she's getting out of that miserable situation,
but ultimately, don't you know she'd rather be happy?
The mind is so powerful—it can entrap us or free us.
But first you have to know you've got the power.

*My power does not frighten me. I*
*own it, and I use it to propel me*
*along my health and fitness*
*program.*

# DAY 296

*Radiant health is a blessing.*

When you're glowing with health, beauty seems to shine forth effortlessly from your body. Health is such a precious gift, we should never take it for granted. Unfortunately, many of us come to appreciate good health when it's too late. It takes our getting sick to realize what a blessing health is, and when the healing finally comes, we can't thank the Creator enough. That's the proper spirit: gratitude. There are so many forces working against the health of our people, from the polluted environment to inferior neighborhood grocery stores to our own inertia. Make a solid commitment today to do something that will bring about healing in body, mind, or spirit.

*My health is so precious I don't want to leave it to chance. I'll eat right, exercise, and make sure to take time to look at a fish and smell the roses.*

*My butt is high. I like where my legs meet my butt—*
*it's quite defined. I can wear almost anything and*
*look good.*
—NAOMI CAMPBELL[26]

Now there's a Black woman with some self-esteem!
Easy, you say, for a model who gets paid in money and
attention for her looks every day. She gets a lot of positive reinforcement. So would you, if you sought it out.
Now if you want self-*worth,* that's different. Naomi gets
a ton of praise from admirers, but does she have self-
worth, the deep inner knowledge of herself as a beautiful spiritual being beyond the external appearance of her
body? Perhaps. Do you? If your self-worth was strong,
you'd be able to say, "My hips roll like the hills. I love
how my legs rub against each other when I walk, creating a sensation of warmth and womanliness in my most
secret place. I can wear any style in any color and look
absolutely fabulous."

*Naomi and I, we love our bodies,*
*and that love comes from a deep*
*inner knowledge that we're*
*incredible.*

# DAY 298

*"Family values" is about health.*

There's been a lot of talk about family values, and unfortunately the term is being used as a whip by politicians and others who would have white women barefoot and pregnant, with Black women serving them and playing mammy to their babies. Today, we take back this perfectly lovely term and restore its original intent. Family values is not about imposing judgment on a family just because the unit doesn't fit the standard husband-wife-2.5 kids model. We understand family values as those life-enhancing beliefs and attitudes that drive the positive day-to-day activities and behaviors of families. Healthy families have healthy values that manifest into healthy lifestyles.

*My family values health, kindness, and truthful communication. We love and respect one another.*

# DAY 299

*Yogurt is womanfood.*

You either love it or you hate it. Try loving yogurt, though. It's got so much of what's good for us, including live friendly bacterial cultures called *Lactobacillus acidophilus* that stimulate the natural flora in the stomach. Not all brands contain the cultures, so make sure you read the labels. Yogurt is low in lactose, which is good news for lactose-intolerant sisters, and it is full of the nutrients women need such as calcium and B-complex vitamins.[27] Yogurt is also great for women who are prone to yeast infections. Eat a cup a day and the yeast just might go away, or at least keep it in check. Plain yogurt is also a great non-fat substitute for cream cheese and sour cream. Instead of eating pre-mixed brands, which usually contain too much sugar, try blending plain non-fat yogurt with fresh fruit, nuts, and honey. Or make a fruit shake. Delicious!

*I'll use my creativity to make yogurt a delicious part of my food program.*

# DAY 300

*America: life, liberty, and the pursuit of fatness.*

*Time* magazine scooped the biggest scandal of the decade. Despite federal government fitness goals, despite new and bigger fitness machines being sold by the millions, despite all the money that has been poured into research, despite all the money we spend on diet club memberships, the country has actually gotten fatter. "According to a report in the *Journal of the American Medical Association,* some 58 million people in the U.S. weigh at least 20% more than their ideal body weight— making them, in the unforgiving terminology of dietary science, obese."[28] So don't feel bad. You're not alone.

 *I may not be alone, but I refuse to stay stuck on fat.*

# DAY 301

*Tomorrow I'll pay for my follies of today.*

Consider the stretch of time that lies ahead of you now. Longevity is often touted as a much desired goal, but what's the point of a long life if your years are wracked with illness and disease and dependency on others? Imagine Methuselah complaining every day for 900 years about his aching back. What a miserable existence! A long, sorry life could be your future lot if you don't take your health seriously today. Medical science can prolong life, maybe indefinitely, but it's up to you to deal with the quality issue.

*As I look into my future, I can see the necessity of creating a healthy lifestyle today to sustain me into my golden years.*

# DAY 302

*Take me to your leader.*

What do you think of when you hear the term "behavior modification?" B. F. Skinner's black box? Pavlov's dogs? *1984* and the New World Order of mind control, brainwashing, and human robots? We know that behavior modification works. To a great extent, we've all been guinea pigs in the black box. Whenever we watch a food commercial then go rummage around in the refrigerator, we've been manipulated. Since we know behavior modification does work, let's take the best that this science has to offer and make it serve our health and fitness efforts. This can be an excellent way to get a grip on unwanted patterns of behavior that have been undermining your program. Behavior modification does not have to be a sinister thing, just so long as its goals and methods are directed by you.

*I will direct my behavior
modification efforts. I'm wise to
the schemes of ad agencies and
others that would try to take me off
my program.*

# DAY 303

*Ooo-wee, baby!*

Ever since the onslaught of AIDS and sexual harassment suits, sex just ain't what it used to be. Celibacy is the latest trend among singles, and even married folks complain about not getting enough good loving. Sex is too good a thing to tuck away in some closet somewhere. Sex is the best thing for body, mind, and soul, not to mention your relationship, since "lite" food. Studies are beginning to confirm what we knew already: Sex is a great aerobic workout that can strengthen the heart. Any kind of exercise is good for the immune system, but good hot sex especially so, because it relieves stress. So by all means, do it in a committed relationship and with a condom.

*Let's get it on!*

# DAY 304

*George Foreman, move over!*

Ever feel like just hitting somebody? Hold it! Before you take out your stress on someone you love, go to a gym instead. Boxing's not just for men anymore. More and more women are putting on the gloves and taking out their frustrations in this male dominated arena. There's something about hitting and punching in a controlled environment that makes you feel good, confident. First you've got to learn the moves: upper cuts, right and left hooks, punches—there's a real science to this sport. It's not just hitting on somebody. Boxing is a healthy way to channel aggression and stress, and it's a great way to get in shape. Invest in a good set of protective gear and gloves, then ask one of the guys to show you the ropes.

*I will dance like a butterfly and
sting like a bee.*

# DAY 305

*What are you thankful for?*

We're not going to wait for a specific day to give thanks. Let's be conscious of projecting an attitude of thankfulness all month. Have you been successful in meeting your health and fitness goals? Even if you're halfway there, you have something to be thankful for. Maybe you're recovering from an illness. Be thankful. Health is such a precious gift. Let us never take it for granted.

*I give thanks for a blessed life and good health.*

# DAY 306

*You eat too fast.* Slow down.
—*YOUR MAMA*

Where's the fire? Why do you eat so fast? The faster you eat, the less likely you'll be able to hear when your body says to stop, it's had enough. Fast eaters tend to eat second and third helpings because they're simply not paying attention to their bodies. They're on automatic pilot. After the first couple of bites, fast eaters seldom taste the food they're eating. Fast eaters also run the risk of overloading their digestive system. Heartburn, nausea, and other symptoms of an upset stomach can occur. All this can be prevented, and you can begin to taste your food, if you'd just slow down. Take small bites and chew well, 15 to 20 times. Chew until the food becomes mush in your mouth.

*I'll slow down. I want to start
tasting my food again.*

# DAY 307

*If you truly loved yourself, what would you do?*

Here's your assignment for today: write up a list of all the things you'd like to do for the pure enjoyment of it. Here's a few ideas to get you started:

- Walk in a warm, summer rain.
- Have hot, protected sex.
- Worship with abandon.
- Dance.
- Sing.
- Take a trip.
- Ride a bike.
- Play volleyball.
- Paint a picture.
- Buy false eyelashes and put them on, then wear them out.
- Go shopping at an upscale thrift shop.
- Cook a scrumptious low-fat gourmet meal.

*I commit to doing one fun thing today.*

# DAY 308

*"Girl, I just gotta have it."*

The next time you get a craving, don't fight it. Instead, imagine yourself eating the whole cake. We usually begin a binge by pretending that we'll only eat one cookie or one tiny sliver of cheesecake or one french fry. We play that game with ourselves, then end up eating the whole thing. We beat ourselves up, we hate ourselves, then we eat some more to deaden the pain, thus beginning a vicious cycle of self-hatred and overeating. If, on the other hand, you imagine yourself eating the whole thing, you'll actually feel a twinge of nausea. Ride with that sick feeling. The more intensely you can see and taste in your imagination, the stronger your reactions will be. Imagination is a powerful tool that can be used to reprogram unwanted behaviors.

*My visualization abilities are powerful. I can actually take control through the conscious use of my imagination.*

# DAY 309

*The bones are holding it all together.*

If it wasn't for the bones in your body, you'd fall completely apart. Your skeletal system is made up of 206 bones, tendons, and ligaments. The skeleton is the structure that supports all your organs and muscles. Bones are tough, flexible, and light. Some bones, like those in the skull, don't move. They exist to protect your brain. Other bones, like those at the elbows or fingers, form joints, and they support the muscles in providing movement. Tendons connect muscles to bones, and ligaments connect dem bones to other bones. To build bone density and prevent osteoporosis, it's important to include calcium rich foods in your diet. If you're worried that you're not getting enough, talk to your doctor or nutritionist about supplements and the right amount that's best for you. And don't forget, weight training is just about the best bone-building exercise for women of any age.[29]

*When my world is threatening to collapse all around me, it's good to know my skeletal system will keep me standing.*

# DAY 310

*MSG stands for More Stupid Garbage.*

Did you know that the purpose of MSG (monosodium glutamate) is to enhance the flavor of food? Can't herbs and spices or chicken stock do that just fine? What's the point of adding a whole lot of dangerous chemicals to our food? Money? Food manufacturers use MSG to fool us into thinking that their products contain more flavor than they do. MSG is a con. This designer chemical has no nutritional value whatsoever. There is nothing natural or good about it. In fact, MSG has been found to cause nervousness, hyperactivity, and irritability in children and adults. The existence of MSG is a sad commentary on the food industry. Please, read labels, and when you order Chinese, tell them "no MSG!"

*MSG is totally unnecessary, possibly dangerous, and I'll make damn sure none of my foods contain a drop of it.*

# DAY 311

*Eat your roughage. I'm not kidding.*
—*Your Mama*

Mama called it roughage; nutritionists today call it fiber. Nature has provided an abundance of fiber sources, including vegetables and grains, to help keep us "regular"—unconstipated, that is. Simple dietary changes can make a world of difference. Don't overcook vegetables, and eat whole-grain breads and brown rice. Impacted colons contain disease-causing toxins that have accumulated over the years. Fiber acts like a broom, sweeping away the dirt and grime of decayed fecal matter. Fiber has also been found to reduce cholesterol levels.

*Once again Mama was right. I'll boost my roughage intake today.*

# DAY 312

*"Girl, these young people come up with the wildest dances."*

The latest craze to hit the dance floor just happens to be a great exercise for toning the entire thigh. It's called the Butterfly, and resembles a pornographic Charleston. Instead of waving your legs from side to side in a happy fashion, butterfly legs flutter slowly and sensuously. Tighten your thighs for maximum toning.

*I'll try this Butterfly, but behind closed doors until I've got it down.*

# DAY 313

*Why are you so hardheaded?*
—*YOUR MAMA*

If you've been hardheaded about working out, don't complain when you can no longer squeeze into that favorite outfit of yours. Like the old folks say, a hard head makes for a soft behind, and a sedentary lifestyle is the surest way to a soft behind. You know the risks: heart disease, osteoporosis, diabetes. With all that you know about health and fitness, there's simply no excuse. You know that Black women lead the nation in obesity and related diseases. You know that children learn from our example.

*I'll stop being so hardheaded, for my health's sake.*

# DAY 314

*Are you wearing your clothes too big?*

Because of the shame associated with being heavy in this skinny-obsessed society, the tendency is for big women to try and hide their bodies. Of course, it never works, but they try anyway. The tent and "muumuu"-style dresses are abominations, a symbol of the heavy woman's shame. Big clothes only make big women look bigger. They're not hiding anything. Not only that, they make big women feel unattractive, unfeminine. Can you imagine sexual beings under those dresses? No way! There may be a woman as passionate as a volcano underneath, but who'd know it? Make sure your clothes fit well—not too tight, not too big. If you need help, there are many speciality stores that now cater exclusively to big women. Ask for help. And throw those muumuus into the garbage.

*I feel so much better when my clothes fit well.*

# DAY 315

*Pinch yourself. Are you dreaming?*

If you've been walking through life half-asleep, half-awake, it's time to shake yourself and wake all the way up. Human robots walk around in a dazed hypnotic state. You're functioning—you're driving the car, caring for kids, getting the work done—but it's as if you're on automatic pilot. People who have been hypnotized are susceptible to all sorts of suggestions. As you walk around in a daze, what are you thinking? What are your thoughts about your body? Are you thinking about candy bars or Long Island Iced Teas? Girl, you've got to snap out of it. You won't be able to change a thing in your life if you're walking around like a zombie, playing the same old mental and emotional programs.

*OK, OK, I'm awake!*

# DAY 316

*We must teach our daughters to love their bodies.*

It's not that we should ignore Black boys, we shouldn't. It's just that our little girls have been woefully neglected. Sociologists know next to nothing about why Black girls are increasingly beginning to act out some of those same negative behaviors displayed by their male peers. The PRIDE 1993–1994 national survey and the 1993 National Household Survey on Drug Abuse reported dramactic increases in marijuana and alcohol use among young Black girls. What's going on? As grandmothers, mothers, cousins, aunts, older sisters, teachers, and mentors, what are we teaching our girls about health—by word and by our own example? We've got to become more conscientious of the example we're setting before our girls. So many changes are occurring in their bodies, they need us to let them know that they're OK and right on schedule.

*My girl is beautiful and smart. For her and myself, I'll model good, healthy behaviors.*

# DAY 317

*Once upon a time . . .*

. . . there was a woman named Portia who had a tendency to wear her sorrows on her body. She was about 5′4″ and weighed 200 pounds. Her family teased her about her heaviness while deliberately withholding praise about her accomplishments. She was the executive director of an agency that helped rescue children from abuse. Portia's sincere devotion to these world-weary children didn't matter to her family. They even chose to ignore her sizable income from her agency salary and real estate investments. One night, as he wiped the thousandth tear from her eyes, her boyfriend said, "Baby, I think they're jealous—your moms, sister, all of 'em." Portia's eyes lit up. This had never occurred to her. "They're jealous of the fact that you make a good living, wear nice clothes, and got a fine, employed Black man who loves you." Portia laughed and wiped her eyes. He was right. They *were* jealous. And that was their problem, not hers, and she decided right then and there that she wasn't going to give a damn about it anymore.

*The moral of the story is: Don't let someone else's feelings, negative or positive, affect how you live your life and feel about yourself.*

# DAY 318

*Let there be light.*
—GOD

There are physical things we can do to raise our energy
levels—eat better, exercise—but here's a prayer to help
raise energy. The Bible says the first thing God did in
creating the universe was speak, and God said, "Let
there be light." Then God's energy, as this wondrous
light, moved to create everything, including us. It took
an enormous amount of energy to do this. To raise your
own energy, pray, "Let there be light—on my body,"
then, "Let there be light in my hair; let there be light in
my face, in my arms, my breasts," right on down to your
toes. See this holy light swirling energetically around
your body. If you do this exercise honestly and rigorously, you will feel your energy level soar. Do not take
this exercise lightly. This is a powerful exercise. Keep
your mind pure while doing it. In fact, if you're upset
or angry, don't do it. Calm yourself first, then begin.

*As I bask in the holy light, I feel
renewed, cleansed, and healthy.*

# DAY 319

*Don't quit!*

Isn't it amazing how season after season Nature fulfills her obligations to grow, to die, and to grow again? Let's learn from Nature's consistency and dependability. Too often we allow our seasons and cycles to interrupt our flow, our momentum. Maintaining a health and fitness program may be easy for you during the summer months, but what about when the rain falls or the cold winds begin to blow? You cannot be any less diligent.

*Rain, sleet, snow, or hail, I will
pursue health and fitness.*

# DAY 320

*Say Amen! to health and fitness.*

Is your faith community committed to the health of its members? One thing that most religions have in common are dietary laws. While they may not be the same from religion to religion, they each share a concern for maintaining the health of the body temple. If your faith community does not have a health ministry, start one. Preach and teach about wellness, fitness, nutrition, disease prevention, stress reduction, and the need to eliminate risky behaviors, like smoking, drinking, and unprotected sex.

*Our bodies are temples. I'll become an evangelist for health.*

# DAY 321

*What is your philosophic approach to life?*

Take this test to determine if you have a basically pessimistic or optimistic approach to life.

1. When you wake up in the morning you sing:
   a. Good morning, sun!
   b. Oh, my aching head.
2. When something bad happens, you say:
   a. I'll just make lemonade out of these lemons.
   b. I don't have any sugar to make the lemonade.

If you checked both A's, you are a basically optimistic person. B answers suggest a no-can-do spirit. Needless to say, a pessimistic approach will not help you in your quest for a healthy, fit body.

*I am an optimist. I know I can achieve my health and fitness goals.*

# DAY 322

*Sit up straight!*
—YOUR MAMA

Your Mother told you to sit up straight, not only because slouching looks bad, but there's something about the physical act of sitting up that builds confidence. A Black woman with a stiffened spine is a wonder to behold. She can do most anything. A straight spine programs resolve and courage to go forth. Any time you feel yourself slouching in faith and hope, take a deep breath and sit up straight.

*My back is straight, and I'm resolved. I can do it!*

# DAY 323

*Do you hear more no's than yes's in your life?*

How many times have you been told no in your life? No to socializing, no to sex, no to your expression of love? Have you learned to say no to yourself as a result? To activities that might be good for you but might be perceived as selfish? To your skills and abilities? To the ability to lose weight or to be at peace at your current weight? Over the course of a lifetime we hear no maybe a million times. Is it any wonder that when we hear yes we don't believe it? To reverse the years of negative effects from hearing no, start today by saying yes to yourself. Can I have some vegetables? Yes! Can I have some water? Yes! Can I run around the block a couple of times? Yes! Can I buy that sharp dress? Definitely! See how easy saying yes can be?

*Being a yes woman is not so bad*
*after all.*

# DAY 324

*Behavioral researchers have estimated that in the
average individual as much as 77% of all our
programs are false.*
—SHAD HELMSTETTER, PH.D.[30]

The mental and emotional programs that drive your behaviors are rooted in childhood, not to mention slavery
experiences. Can you imagine most of them being bad
for you? That means we all need to reevaluate our beliefs. We are all ultimately responsible for our behaviors,
but your bad programming may be undermining your
best efforts to make yourself healthy and fit. You may
need help to find out what they are.

*I'm going to unravel those bad
programs and replace them with
life-affirming ones.*

# DAY 325

*Keep the lips zipped.*

Try this exercise from *Self-Talk for Weight Loss* today: say not one word about food, not one word *all day*.[31] (Of course, if you want to go longer, feel free.) You'll be amazed at how much food has become an obsession. Food is on the brain day and night, what to eat, whether to eat, how much. We even dream about food. For today at least, let's shut our mouths and ruthlessly deal with food thoughts.

*Instead of talking about food, I'll pray for strength.*

# DAY 326

Stay safe. No matter where in the world you live, there will be risks. And few things are worse to your physical and emotional health than an attack. Secure your doors and windows with decorative iron bars. Make sure you lock your car doors when you're either inside or outside the car. In fact, when you're approaching your car, be aware of your environment. Look around. Look under the car and in the back seat. Keep your purse on the floor, out of sight. It's a sad fact of life in the twentieth century, but you must take precautions, and you must teach safety to your children.

*I won't take unnecessary chances
with my life.*

# DAY 327

*"If melanin's such a big deal, why didn't we learn about it in high school biology class?"*

Melanin is the one chemical we Black women have in abundance, but know next to nothing about. We know that melanin colors our skin and protects us from the sun's ultra-violet rays, but there's so much more to it than that. Are you aware of the aggressive research that's being conducted in labs all over the world on this black chemical? Researcher Carol Barnes says that melanin helps us in memory retrieval, immunity against cancer, motor development, and even intuition.[32] Melatonin tablets, melanin treated sunglasses—all kinds of new products are being developed based on the new discoveries. We've got it free of charge. No wonder we're such a natural, jazzy people.

*I am thankful to be blessed with an abundance of melanin.*

# DAY 328

*What's eating you?*

Here's an exercise that will help you discover some of
the unconscious ideas that are keeping you miles from
your goal. Say to yourself the most outrageous affirma-
tion you can think of, like, "I am the most magnificent
woman ever born." Now, quickly, write down every
objection that comes to heart and mind. There will
probably be many, from "I don't believe it" to "Loquisha's body is in much better shape than mine." That's
OK. We often relegate negative thoughts to the back
burner, but they're always a presence in our lives, undermining our best intentions. We need to know what
they are so that we can defeat them and get on with the
business of health.

*I really am extraordinarily
incredible.*

# DAY 329

*Talk is cheap—talk TV, that is.*

Why are we Black women allowing ourselves to be exploited on TV talk shows? Our trials and tribulations have provided grist for the talk mill; damn near every problem facing our community has been laid bare to titillate and excite millions of people. We hear the most uncomfortably intimate conversations. We used to be such a private people; family matters were kept within the family. Today, though, our privacy has become a commodity that we sell cheap for travel expenses. How many of us cringe when some sister fights with another over a man who's fathered eleven children by ten women? Or when heavy women feel the need to defend their wearing of sexy clothes before a skinny-oriented public. We feel their pain and embarrassment. These intimate portraits serve none of us, men, women, or our children. Yes, our community is facing serious problems, and yes, we need to talk *amongst ourselves*. Let's come together and work them out.

*We don't have to be buffoons*
*before a leering public.*

# DAY 330

*Flo Jo's weight loss secret: If you attach an extraordinary goal to the desire for weight loss, you increase your chances of success.*

Would the goal of an Olympic gold medal be high enough to motivate you to work out and eat right? When Olympic medalist (three golds, one silver in 1988) Florence Griffith gained 65 pounds during her pregnancy, she knew she was going to have to reach for the stars to get back into running shape. Her motto was, "If I don't buy it, I won't try it. And if I don't fry it, I won't have to diet."[33] During the training season, Flo Jo follows a vegetarian eating program. With her intense training schedule she can afford to splurge occasionally on ice cream, french fries, and a slice of lower-fat sweet potato pie, but she doesn't let the cravings get the best of her. Her goal of a gold medal in 1996 is motivating enough to keep her on track.

*Flo Jo and I know how to run this race and win.*

# DAY 331

*Don't panic!*

We all blow it at one time or another. Feasting days like
Thanksgiving are tough on our resolve, and we're not
always successful in practicing moderation. Don't beat
yourself up if you backslide a bit. Don't allow one set-
back to ruin your entire effort. Just get back on the program. You can do this.

*I will love myself through the
disappointments.*

# DAY 332

*When was the last time you felt completely and totally loved?*

We Black women love our men so completely and deeply that we often relegate equally important loves to the periphery. But we all long for an unconditional love that accepts us for who and why we are who we are. Our children love us that way. They love purely and unconditionally. Let's learn to love ourselves with the purity and intensity of a child. And let's learn to move all sources of love front and center, right where it truly belongs.

*Loving myself must be equally important as loving someone else.*

# DAY 333

*Are you allergic to your mate?*

A myth is a story or event that may or may not be true. There is a psychological myth floating around that says that men fare much better health-wise in marriage than in bachelorhood. Women, on the other hand, don't do so well in marriage, and unless they have close women friends, they are at risk of sickness and a shortened life. Statistics are used to support this assertion. What is this saying, that men are bad for our health? Do we believe this? Sure, we get pissed off at the brethren from time to time, but isn't this a bit extreme? Or is it? Even though male-female relationship discussions can get pretty heated, maybe this is something we need to talk about.

*I'm not going to believe everything I hear. Besides, if my mate is making me sick, and I'm still with him, what does that say about me?*

# DAY 334

*Reclaim your dreams.*

What do you want to be when you grow up? Remember how we used to answer that question? We would try to imagine ourselves in the most glamorous jobs. Even stuffing envelopes seemed exciting back then. Unfortunately, for too many of us, life got in the way of our dreams, and we settled for boring, monotonous jobs. There is nothing worse than waiting for five o'clock to come. How do you pass the time on your job? How do you handle the stress that comes from feeling unfulfilled in work? Are you nibbling throughout the day? Have you become sedentary in the evenings because work has so completely stressed you out? Consider this: some of your weight gain might be job related. Full-time employees spend one-third of their days on the job. If you hate your work, then one-third of your day will be spent doing things that cause you great anguish. If this is your life, then it's time for a change. It's time to embark on the greatest quest facing the Black woman: discovering your life's mission. Getting to know your mission will require much prayer and soul searching, but once you discover it, food will lessen in importance.

*I will be anything I dare and
dream to be!*

# DAY 335

*Happy birthday to us all!*

Although the celebration of Jesus' birth is a Christian one, we can all learn from His life during the holiday season, regardless of our faith or creed. Jesus taught us wonderful lessons in giving, forgiveness, love (especially self-love), service, justice, and compassion. These are characteristics we should all seek to birth in our new healthy selves. If we all abided by these simple concepts, the world would be a healthier, saner place. Imagine healed Black communities where people actually loved each other, looked out for one another, showed each other mercy and compassion. We'd be a different type of people.

*It is always the season to pray the healing spirit into our communities.*

# DAY 336

*Give of yourself.*

When Christmas rolls around this season, try not to overspend. Instead, spend some time at a homeless shelter. Or offer a single parent friend some baby-sitting hours. Senior citizen homes are filled with lonely people, especially during this time of year. Pay an elder a visit. There are some poor children in your very own neighborhood who have never received a Christmas present. If anyone should get a teddy bear and a hug, they should, and you should give it to them.

*I will give of my time this season—
just because it's the right thing
to do.*

# DAY 337

*Got those holiday blues?*

Have you ever wanted to wail a few laments on a saxophone during the holiday season? Just how much festivity and joy to the world can one woman stand? The year-end holidays can be a rough time, not just for Black women, but everybody. Some of us are mourning a difficult year. Others are lonely for family, friends, or that special someone. If you haven't yet achieved your goals or received your heart's desire, this gift-giving season falls flat. "Why me?" is a popular blues refrain sung by sad women. If you're one of the many in this country who tend to become depressed during the holiday season, take comfort in knowing that you're not alone. That's why it's so important to be kind to yourself. Don't beat yourself up for what you're feeling, and please, go easy on the alcohol. Besides being loaded with calories, you don't want to compound your problems with a new addiction. How about taking a trip to an exotic island? If you can't afford to get away, volunteer for a children's program or some other worthy cause. Helping others gets your mind off your problems, and you'll feel so much better afterward.

*I'm going to grit my teeth and get through this. Besides, life's not so bad. In fact, apart from this holiday madness, life's pretty darn good.*

# DAY 338

*Let there be peace on earth, and let it begin in me.*

Wars and rumors of wars. Mean-spirited public debates. Black women and Black men at each other's throats. The widening gap between the generations. Looks like we've got two options: (1) Either we take individual responsibility for creating peace in our lives, and thus, peace in the world, or (2) Mama Earth is going to start kicking butt. Can you imagine what a peaceful life would be like? (And don't mistake boredom for peace.) Peace = calm. You know that peace is reigning when you can smile even when you're standing in the midst of chaos. Peace = harmony. Work to integrate all aspects of your multifaceted self. Let's harmonize our communities. Peace = health. It's very difficult to maintain health when you're stressed out all the time.

*Peace begins at my address.*

# DAY 339

*Connect what you know to what you do.*

If we're so smart, how come we keep on doing the same dumb stuff? We know we're supposed to exercise, drink water, and cut down on fat and calories, yet we keep putting it off until Monday. Repeat positive messages over and over during the course of the day. Post messages on your wallet, bedside table, refrigerator, mirror, computer. Repetition strengthens new mental programs. The more you think a thing, the more likely you are to commit action to it.

*I know a lot about health and fitness now, and I'm going to prove it. I'm going to apply what I know to my everyday behavior.*

# DAY 340

*Grown women should never allow their emotions to get the best of them.*

Are you a woman, or are you a mouse? Emotions can make a woman out of you, or they can keep you in a childlike state. Psychologists say that the way we emotionally respond to situations was learned in adolescence. In other words, you're probably still acting the way you did when you were twelve years old! When you're depressed, do you eat yourself into a trance? When you get mad at your man, do you throw his clothes out the window? Your emotions are valid; however, it's time to learn new, healthy ways of dealing with them.

*I'm going to start acting like a grown-up.*

# DAY 341

*What do you want out of life?*

Big question! What's your ultimate dream? Give yourself the gift of believing that what you desire can become a reality. Learn how to believe in the impossible again. Don't let the disappointments of life distract you from achieving your goal. You don't want to look back on your life and regret most of it. The worst regret in life is not even having tried. Use this month to begin planning how you will make some of those old dreams a reality.

*I'm not afraid to dream big. I'm a*
*Black woman, and I have the*
*power to make it happen.*

# DAY 342

*Snack strategically.*

Snacks have gotten a bad rap because we tend to use them for oral gratification rather than nutritional sustenance and energy boosters. Don't waste valuable snack calories on high-fat coffee cakes and sweet rolls. Not only will they go directly to your thighs, they'll give you a fake high. You feel better for a moment, but inevitably you'll crash. Heavy women have a bad reputation for nonstop snacking, but possibly all that eating might have more to do with trying to restore depleted energy reserves than gluttony. Snack on fresh fruit, low-fat bran muffins, celery sticks, and wheat crackers.

*I will snack more wisely.*

# DAY 343

*Give loved ones the gift of health.*

If you buy gifts, make them healthy ones. No more fruit cakes. (Does anyone eat that stuff?) No more video games, no more alcohol. Buy motivational tapes and books for loved ones. Roller skates, basketballs, and jump ropes will be treasured by kids. How about a free membership to a walking club that you're about to create? Gym shoes, sweats, dumbbells, mini trampolines. The ideas are endless. Low-fat cookbooks, a subscription to a health and fitness magazine, this book . . .

*Even if they're not thinking about health and fitness, I'm going to give it to them anyway!*

# DAY 344

*Inside every one of us lurks a wild woman struggling to break free.*

Josephine Baker, Grace Jones, Chaka Khan, Salt 'N Peppa. These are our wild women, and we love them, envy them, and sometimes fear for their lives. They live life at the edge and beyond, and societal norms be damned. There are no cages around their fired-up personalities. They are free to express and create according to the dictates of their inner promptings. Josephine Baker was a scandalous woman who broke all the rules as she performed half nude in banana skirts throughout the theaters of Europe. Salt 'N Peppa's experimentation with outrageous rap poetry and wild hairstyles and clothes resonates with the rebelliousness of an entire generation. We may talk about these wild women behind their backs, but secretly, many of us wish we felt as free and unbound by rules and responsibilities. We might not want to be as extreme as our wild sisters, but we can learn from them. Every once in a while, do something outrageous. Wear some really red lipstick, or get that fly haircut you've been thinking about. Show off your legs. It's healthy to break free of routines and just go party.

*My wild woman's going to get a breath of fresh air today.*

# DAY 345

*Love yourself unconditionally.*

Who loves ya, babe? If no one else does (which is hard to believe, you're so cute), *you've* got to love you, and without reservation. Give yourself the gift of a complete spa treatment—get a massage, manicure, facial—the works! Loving yourself means ending all destructive relationships. Lighten your load for the new year. Get rid of the dead weight in your life. Loving yourself means surrounding yourself with beauty. Buy a flower for the kitchen table. Put out the candles and the good china. Loving yourself means exercising and eating nutritiously.

*Loving myself is such an easy thing to do.*

# DAY 346

*It's time for the Sleeping Giant to awaken.*

Black people in America are often called the Sleeping Giant—sleeping, because too many of us are passive about the oppressive conditions in which we live; giant, because even though we're in the minority in this country, our numbers are great. When we finally wake up, we'll be a force to be reckoned with. Until then, we'll continue to live under conditions that diminish the quality of life for ourselves and our children. How long will we continue to be passive about the waste dumps, toxic factory air, and unclean water in our communities? How long will we continue to allow other people to come into our communities and sell us stale food and an abundance of liquor? How long will we passively accept the existence of drug dealers who deal dope to our children? Why are we so passive about our health? What are we waiting for?

*Sleeping Giant, this is your wake-up call.*

# DAY 347

*Take off the kid gloves.*

Become a no-limit woman. Don't let racism, sexism, capitalism, socialism, conservatism, liberalism, or religion put a ceiling on your dreaming. Try this exercise: When it turns dark, go outside and look straight up. See those stars? There lie your goals. Imagine a perfectly healthy body. No aches, no pains. Imagine yourself totally free from food obsession. Whatever you want, you can have. All you have to do is believe, and work diligently to achieve your goals.

*I have the courage to dream
big dreams.*

# DAY 348

*Is your relationship based on the body?*

A woman told her fiancé, "Honey, do you find me attractive even though I have this stomach?" Now the woman had a normal woman's body—curvy in all the right places, serious hips, and a nicely rounded stomach. The man told her to do some sit-ups, and everything would be fine. But suppose she gets caught up in the wedding preparations and doesn't have time for sit-ups? Will they be able to enjoy their wedding night? Will she end up feeling badly about her body? Do you think her self-worth will make it through this challenge? How long will these two stay married? For love to last, the body business has got to be incidental. Marriage is about two human beings coming together—not two bodies. Before you tie the knot, make sure both of your priorities are in order.

*I am a spiritual being who just
happens to inhabit this body.*

# DAY 349

*Never again.*

When a people make a conscious decision not to repeat the past they say, "Never again." The Jews have annual ceremonies to remind the world that they will never let the death camps happen again. They remind us over and over of the events of the past. Black people, on the other hand, want to forget slavery and Jim Crow. It's as if we've been fully integrated into American society. No one admits to racism anymore, and because we're so anxious to forget the past, the forces of evil are getting away with murder. Again. If we choose to forget, we'll keep making the same mistakes over and over. With courage and purpose we must periodically revisit the past, not to dwell there or be victimized by it, but to learn from it.

*Never again will I forget the
lessons of the past.*

# DAY 350

*Take time to reflect on your accomplishments of the past year.*

Take a few moments to think back on your past twelve months. It wasn't all bad, was it? In fact, you did a lot of good things. Get out a sheet of paper and write down all the good stuff that you did, or that happened to you. How did you help others? Did you make real progress on your health and fitness plan? Did you earn a promotion? Win a citation? Help a little old lady across the street? No matter how small, write it down. Whenever you feel down, pull out the sheet of paper and rejoice.

*I'm not so bad after all. In fact, I'm pretty good!*

# DAY 351

*It's time to clean house.*

How healthy is your colon? The answer to that question may help explain a lot of problems that we who live in this meat-eating, junk food imbibing society are having with our bodies. The colon is a five-foot long tube through which all the stuff that we've ingested—from food to booze to drugs—passes through and out of the body. Problems occur, however, when, for whatever reason, that stuff gets stuck in the colon. When the walls of the colon become impacted with fecal matter, the body's resistance to disease is weakened. Impacted, decaying fecal matter is poison to the body, causing a wide range of maladies, from gas and constipation to colon cancer. A diet high in fiber, that is, fresh fruits, vegetables, beans, etc., will help, but sometimes colonics are needed to cleanse the colon thoroughly. Ask around for a good practitioner and don't be put off by the procedure. It only takes about a half-hour, and the discomfort is minimal.

*A little dirty business is well worth
the health of my body.*

# DAY 352

*Let's say you did have the money for cosmetic surgery.
Would you do it?*

You can have your cellulite vacuumed out of your
thighs, or you can get your breasts lifted. How about a
face-lift or a tummy tuck? Or are you one of those
women who believe that if God had intended for you
to have perky breasts He would have kept you sixteen
years old? It's a deep thing, this cosmetic surgery. Look
at what Michael Jackson did. He's an extreme case, but
what an interesting question he raises. For Black
women, can cosmetic surgery ever be just about beau-
tification, or will there always be racial overtones to consider? Another question: have you ever known a white
woman to make her nose bigger?

*I'm so gorgeous, cosmetic surgery
would be a waste of time. I think
I'll invest my money in real estate
instead.*

# DAY 353

*Black power, baby!*

What is Black power? The term, popular in the 1960s, was the collective rallying cry for a people who had been under tremendous oppression for much too long. It was an empowering slogan, so why don't we say it anymore, throwing our fists high in the air for emphasis? Has our Black power been defused? Who pulled the plug on our Black power? Physicists tell us that energy is never destroyed, only recycled into other forms. Take heart, our power survives. Individually, we have the power to build healthy lives. Together, we can build healthy communities. A wonderful Black power exercise is to stand outside and imagine the melanin in your skin drawing the sun's rays into your body. If you can do this with friends, family, coworkers, or faith sisters and brothers, so much the better. As you soak up the energy of the sun, know that individually and collectively we are powerhouses of health, beauty, wisdom, and productive action.

*Today I use my thoughts to direct
the flow of my Black power into
productive endeavors.*

# DAY 354

*Janet's grandmother used to say that she was just carrying around baby fat, but as far as Janet was concerned, "It was never baby fat . . . just fat."*[34]

When Janet Jackson commands the stage, everyone, male and female, gasps at the perfection of her African woman body. To look at her now, you'd never imagine that she was a plump child. Whether her grandmother's categorization of fat as "baby fat" contributed to body image problems during later years, we don't know, but if Janet's anything like the rest of us, probably so. The way we feel about our bodies today began in girlhood. There is one, and only one, acceptable body type, and Lord help the 99 percent of us who don't conform. Understand your personal history, and you'll begin to unravel some of the mysteries of your eating behavior. Also, reinforce your daughter's sense of her physical beauty *and* intelligence. Be her model of exercise and a healthy lifestyle. Listen to her carefully and nip that bad programming in the bud.

*As I understand my unconscious motivations, I become less susceptible to old, useless programs.*

# DAY 355

*Self-love means self-acceptance.*

You can't love anyone you don't accept, and that goes for yourself. Even as you're working to change your life and your body, you must still maintain a basic acceptance of who you are. After all, you're not trying to change the wondrous essence of you. People who do that are doomed to failure, because their past will always return to haunt them. You can change your name, your address, even your face and hair color, but you cannot change that spirit that makes you *you*. The quicker you're able to come to peace with that fact, the quicker you'll be able to make real progress in your quest for a healthy body.

*The Creator accepts me just as I am, and who am I to question that judgment? I accept and love myself.*

# DAY 356

*How are you spending your time during the
holiday season?*

For some of us it's feast, and for others it's famine. Either you love that time of the year, or you can't wait until it's all over. Stress and depression are common. Others love the partying and all the hoopla. Regardless, don't forget that moments alone can help regenerate your spirit and remind you of the true purpose of the season. The best gift you can give yourself is daily peace and quiet. Take time out for yourself. Peace time is absolutely essential for your sanity.

*Quality time is the gift I will give
to myself during the holiday season.*

# DAY 357

*Give yourself a gift of positive thought.*

It's how you think that counts. Just for today, no matter what happens, think on a high plane. Today you have no enemies, you have no worries. Your life is a precious gift. Think not one harsh thought against your body. Bless your hair, your beautiful face, your breasts, stomach, behind, and legs. Bless your life and the lives of your loved ones. Wear a smile. Glow like the sun, or a star. That's right, all day. You can do it.

*You know, I really do feel happy
today.*

# DAY 358

*Oh, Mary, don't you weep.*
*—NEGRO SPIRITUAL*

Oh, the pain of delivering a new life! Is there anything
quite like it? Camille Cosby said it's like pulling your
bottom lip over your entire head. But when the baby
comes, the miracle and beauty of that tiny being far out-
weighs the pain you've suffered. If you want to birth a
new life for yourself, don't expect it to be easy. There
may be some pain and suffering. There may be some discomfort. But the miracle and beauty of your new life will
be worth all the trials and tribulations you've endured.
Changing your lifestyle to birth a new body is one of the
greatest challenges you can ever set for yourself. Already
you've demonstrated courage and a noble desire to stop
complaining and do something about it. That's a big,
bold step in the right direction.

*Mary birthed a divine Being into*
*the world. As a Black woman, I*
*also have the power to create*
*miracles in my life.*

# DAY 359

*Kwanzaa:* Umoja *means unity.*

Let's take a lesson from the days of Kwanzaa. There's inspiration, motivation, and safety in numbers. Form a walking club at work or on your block. Don't spend any money on expensive equipment or fancy clothes. Just wear some comfortable sweats and a good pair of gym shoes, and hit the street. As you're walking, remind each other to hold in your stomachs, breathe rhythmically, and take long strides. Bend your arms and pump 'em up. We've always been at our best and accomplished the most when we practiced umoja.

*I will get together with my health-conscious friends.*

# DAY 360

*Kwanzaa:* Kujichagulia *means self-determination.*

The twentieth century has been a trip for Black people. There have been two forces at war among us: the liberationists and the accommodationists. The liberationists fight for freedom from oppression and assume the right to determine the quality, shape, and character of their lives for themselves. The accommodationists beg for trinkets and opportunities and apologies. Liberationists and accommodationists can be found in all camps—liberal, conservative, Democrat, and Republican. We choose to side with the liberationists. When it comes to the health of our communities, we will determine how *we* will care for the sick and elderly among us. *We'll* decide how and what to eat. Food establishments selling death in our neighborhoods have got to go. Health, which directly correlates to intellectual development, vitality, longevity, and overall quality of life, is now a priority. This we decide for ourselves.

*Kujichagulia is a powerful concept
and I will meditate it into my
spirit and actions.*

# DAY 361

*Kwanzaa:* Ujima *means collective work and responsibility.*

To clean up the health tragedy in our communities, we're all going to have to pull together—the faith communities, businesses, activists, politicians, schools, families, media, agencies, and individuals. We've got to create safe places where our children can go out and play. They need fresh air and exercise; so many are woefully out of shape. We've got to care more about the nutritional needs of our elderly. Too many of them are malnourished and alone. We ourselves have got to work together to regain health and vitality. It'll be hard work, but we can do it if we come together and share the responsibility for healing our communities. We've got to remember the feel and shape of community. Within that word *community* is "unity."

*We Black women have never been afraid of hard work. We've got the ujima spirit.*

# DAY 362

*Kwanzaa:* Ujamaa *means cooperative economics.*

Getting healthy and fit doesn't have to cost you an arm and a leg. Sometimes we feel overwhelmed by it all because we try to go it alone, but if we pool our money, we can get much more accomplished. Here are some ways you and your friends can pool resources to make your fitness program more fun and effective:

1. Collective buying can save you money. Your local health club may give your group a discount if you join together.
2. Form a food cooperative, and you'll be able to buy fresh produce and other items wholesale.
3. Hire a personal trainer to work out with a group of you in your home.
4. Pool money to buy good exercise equipment.

*I don't want to do this alone. I can economize by pooling my resources with friends and family.*

# DAY 363

*Kwanzaa:* Nia *means purpose.*

A Black woman with purpose is a Black woman on a mission. She has little time for risky behaviors. She is focused, more or less content, busy and not always looking at the clock. How do you find your purpose in life? When you begin to ask yourself burning questions like, "Who am I?" and "Why am I here?" then you're on the threshold of discovery. Many people have found their purpose by remembering their childhood passions and hobbies. Others have embarked on deep spiritual quests to obtain divine revelations.

*Good health is a bigger issue than just my body. I am a woman with a purpose.*

# DAY 364

*Kwanzaa:* Kuumba *means creativity.*

Black women are some of the most creative people on the planet. We sing, we dance, we cook, we sew, and we make love in such unique ways. We are watched and studied by the world. Our ways are often stolen and exploited, but that has never stopped us from creating and dreaming. We still keep stepping to our own beat. We are amazing, wonderful, beautiful, creative Black women.

*My time on earth will be meaningful. My life will be a creative experience of joy, love, and health.*

# DAY 365

*Kwanzaa:* Imani *means faith.*

For so long we have depended on the faith of our mothers to pull us through the trials of life. Now we've got to stand on our own and work our faith as rigorously as we work out our bodies. Faith is like a muscle. You've got to exercise it to make it strong. The elders talk a lot about "stepping out on faith." It's an act of courage to step out when you don't see how your dream can possibly happen. Faith is the unwavering belief in ourselves to get a job done. Women of faith believe that a kind and generous universe will help them. Every turn of the corner, every walk down the street holds the potential for manifestation. Women of faith have an air of expectancy, and they've learned the virtue of patience. Planning lays the foundation for change in our lives, action moves us forward, and faith is the glue that connects the plan to the end result.

*Today I become a faith woman. I believe in my power to manifest.*

# NOTES

1. page 28 – Bikram Choudhury, *Bikram's Beginning Yoga Class* (New York: G. P. Putnam's Sons, 1978), p. 13.

2. page 44 – Rachael F. and Richard F. Heller, *The Carbohydrate Addict's Diet* (New York: Penguin Group, 1991).

3. page 61 – *Steppin'* is a highly stylized form of Black dance that has a long-standing tradition in Chicago and other urban cities. Some call it Black ballroom dancing. Couples improvise intricate steps together to rhythm and blues tunes, usually from the 1960s and 1970s. A *steppers set* is a dance party.

4. page 77 – Stephen Blauer, *The Juicing Book* (Garden City Park, New York: Avery Publishing Group Inc., 1989), pp. 87–88.

5. page 90 – Deborah Gregory, "The Queen Rules: Regal Queen Latifah Rules Her Hip-Hop Empire with Flavor, B-Women Business Skill and a Little Help from Mom," *Essence,* October 1993, p. 56.

6. page 98 – *Healthy People 2000: National Health Promotion and Disease Prevention Objectives,* published by U.S. Department of Health and Human Services and Public Health Service, Centers for Disease and Prevention, 1994.

7. page 109 – David Salariya and Kathryn Senior, *The X-Ray Picture Book of Your Body* (Chicago: Franklin Watts, 1993), pp. 16–17.

8. page 119 – U.S. Department of Commerce, Economic and Statistics Administration, Bureau of the Census, *Statistical Abstract of the United States,* 1994.

9. page 120 – Linda Villarosa, ed., *Body & Soul: The Black Women's Guide to Physical Health and Emotional Well-Being* (New York: HarperPerennial, 1994), p. 321.

10. page 128 – *Healthy People 2000: National Health Promotion and Disease Prevention Objectives,* U.S. Department of Health

and Human Services and Public Health Service Centers for Disease and Prevention, 1994.

**11.** page 161 – Patricia Fisher, ed., *Age Erasers for Women: Actions You Can Take Right Now to Look Younger and Feel Great* (Emmaus, Penn.: Rodale Press, 1994), pp. 256–57.

**12.** page 169 – Tom Monte, *Staying Young: How to Prevent, Slow or Reverse More Than 60 Signs of Aging* (Emmaus, Penn.: Rodale Press, 1994), p. 177.

**13.** page 171 – "Take Control of Monthly Moodiness," *McCall's,* March 1995, p. 44.

**14.** page 174 – Russell Wild, ed., *The Complete Book of Natural & Medicinal Cures* (Emmaus, Pennsylvania: Rodale Press, 1994), p. 80.

**15.** page 180 – "A Woman of Substance," *Women's Sports & Fitness,* January/February 1995, p. 22.

**16.** page 187 – Estella Conwill Majozo, "Milk Children," a poem from *Jiva Telling Rites* (Chicago: Third World Press, 1991), p. 41.

**17.** page 191 – Rosie Daley, *In the Kitchen with Rosie: Oprah's Favorite Recipes* (New York: Alfred A. Knopf, 1994), pp. 39–40.

**18.** page 196 – Lisa Klugman, "The Best Bodies in Hollywood," *New Body* (February 1995), p. 26.

**19.** page 204 – "Cran-'berry' good for you!" *First,* 5 February, 1995, p. 22.

**20.** page 205 – *The Complete Book of Natural and Medicinal Cures* (Emmaus, Penn.: Rodale Press, 1994), p. 77.

**21.** page 207 – Aldore D. Collier, "Singer Vesta Tells How She Lost Almost 100 Pounds," *Jet,* 6 February, 1995, p. 31.

**22.** page 209 – Elizabeth Somer, M.A., R.D., "The Lowdown on Iron," *Shape,* June 1993, p. 38.

**23.** page 225 – Dick Gregory, *Dick Gregory's Natural Diet for Folks Who Eat: Cookin' with Mother Nature* (New York: Harper and Row, 1973), p. 3.

24. page 252 – *Home Remedies Just for Women: Doctor-Proven Tips & Techniques for Everyday Health Problems* (Emmaus, Penn.: Rodale Press, 1994), pp. 25–26.

25. page 285 – Professor Leonard Jeffries, lecture given at Kennedy King, Jr. College, Chicago, White Supremacy Conference, October 1990.

26. page 297 – Lisa Klugman, "The Best Bodies in Hollywood," *New Body*, February 1995, p. 27.

27. page 299 – Russell Wild, ed. *The Complete Book of Natural & Medicinal Cures* (Emmaus, Penn.: Rodale Press, 1994), p. 108.

28. page 300 – Philip Elmer-Dewitt, "Fat Times," *Time*, 16 January, 1995, p. 59.

29. page 309 – David Salariya and Kathryn Senior, *The X-Ray Picture Book of Your Body* (Chicago: Franklin Watts, 1993), p. 8.

30. page 324 – Shad Helmstetter, Ph.D., *Self-Talk for Weight Loss: Lose Weight, Keep It Off, and Never Diet Again* (River Productions, Inc., 1994), p. 21.

31. page 325 – Shad Helmstetter, Ph.D., *Self-Talk for Weight Loss: Lose Weight, Keep It Off, and Never Diet Again* (River Productions, Inc., 1994), p. 110.

32. page 327 – Carol Barnes, *Melanin: The Chemical Key to Black Greatness* (Houston, TX: C. B. Publishers, 1988), p. 55.

33. page 330 – Lisa C. Jones, "How to Splurge on Holiday Goodies without Getting Fat," *Ebony*, December 1994, p. 65.

34. page 354 – Lynn Norment, "Grown-Up Janet Jackson," *Ebony*, September 1993, p. 42.